Two Steps Forward, One Step Back

~A Journey Through Life~ Ulcerative Colitis and the Specific Carbohydrate Diet™

Tucker Sweeney

&

Carol Thompson

Published by Tucker Sweeney

Bonners Ferry, ID 83805

Printed by CreateSpace

Edited by Donna Coombs, Dan Cullinane, Jim Reason, Carol Thompson, Katie Sweeney, Dylan Sweeney, and Tucker Sweeney.

First Printing September 2011

ISBN-13: 978-1466201804

ISBN-10: 1466201800

Photography: Tucker Sweeney, Kale Semar, Aaron Hanson. Permission granted.

Cover photo: Kale Semar. Climbing in the Sierras, CA

Back cover photo: Stephanie Butler.

Disclaimer:

The information, opinions, and content in this book are for educational purposes only. It is not intended to replace the advice of a physician or medical practitioner. Please see your health care provider before beginning any new health program.

Specific Carbohydrate Diet and SCD are trademarks of Kirkton Press Limited

Table of Contents

Table of Contents

Recipes

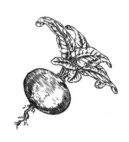

6

Acknowledgments

Throughout this journey there have been so many people who have helped me along the way. I would like to thank my grandparents, Peg and Paul for your help and understanding of the SCD and helping to facilitate a discovery of health through cooking adventures and inquisitive questioning.

Thanks go out to Grandma Sue for letting me fill your kitchen with yogurt makers, pots and pans filled with SCD cooking, and multiple dishwasher loads. Also, thank you for connecting me with others who are afflicted with UC and who follow the diet.

Thank you to Grandpa Wayne, a retired doctor, for reading through the many medical research papers and helping us to understand them.

I wouldn't be writing this book or in such good health if it wasn't for Don Trosset, who told me about the SCD and answered many of my questions in the beginning. Thank you so much for taking the time to share information with me that potentially saved my life.

Lucy Rosset is another person who is tightly connected to the SCD and answered many of my questions early on. Thank you for taking the time to listen, encourage, and be a wealth of information.

I would personally like to thank my parents and family for all that you did during many hard years. Dad, thank you for keeping me optimistic during such a bleak period in my life and for taking the time to listen and research alternative methods to combat my ailment. Thank you to Jodi for being so innovative in your cooking and for taking the time to prepare things that I could eat; sometimes being the only one to think of it during family gatherings. It means a lot and you and Joe are amazing at what you do.

To Anna Phillips, Spud, and the Bricker family it means the world to me the understanding and support you give to Katie and I, the SCD, and for all that you prepare when we visit during the holidays. It really helps and makes this all work. Thank you.

To my Mom and Steve: you have been like a rock from start to finish in this wild life. Steve, you have always been supportive of my dietary restrictions, as well as the time certain things require. Thank you. Mom, wow where to begin? You took the bull by the horns with the SCD and you made it work, start to finish. You were supportive, comforting, strong, and insightful, and I cannot thank you enough. You worked tirelessly when I had almost given up, and without you I really don't know if this all would have worked out like it did. Also, without you I most likely would not have decided to write a book like this. You saw the need, took it upon yourself to see it through, and here we are with a finished copy! You're a superstar!

To Dylan, thanks for being such a supportive and understanding brother when it came to me being sick. Not only did you give me the time I needed while putting your needs aside, you also helped me to feel normal during such trying times. Thanks, bro.

To my friends Kale, Winter, Aaron, Lewis, Andrew, Lori, and countless others. Thank you for being the great and understanding people you are. Whether it was packing pounds of raw hamburger through bear territory, hauling coolers full of fresh vegetables through airports, or just being there to listen during a rough time in my life, thank you.

I would like to extend a big thank you to Donna, Dan, and Jim for looking over the book and putting considerable time into editing it. Writing this book was only half the battle and you helped make it what it is today. Thank you.

Lastly, I would like to thank my beautiful wife Katie. You brought the sun when there were clouds and you gave me peace when there was chaos. As a spouse you understood and respected the turmoil that I confronted on a daily basis and gave me the strength to carry on. You cared for me and looked at who I was minus the disease, for which I will forever be grateful. I love you, respect you, and can't wait to cook with you night after night. To Pepper…Get em!

Foreword

By Katie Sweeney

I write this foreword from a unique standpoint in Tucker's life. I am his wife, a nurse by occupation, and finishing my degree as a family nurse practitioner. Ulcerative colitis has affected my life in more ways than I can count. I first encountered the disease when my father told me he was diagnosed with "an ulcer from stress and drinking too much coffee".

I was in my first year of nursing school when he fell very ill with weight loss and all of the many horrible symptoms that accompany ulcerative colitis. At the time I had never heard of ulcerative colitis, but as I watched my father deteriorate as a result of this disease, I had to beg him to let me drive him to the hospital. He was given only one option of surgery, because his colon was so far damaged. The doctors said that if he had waited any longer he might have died.

Being a nurse, a daughter, and a wife, I can truly and honestly tell you that men are great procrastinators when it comes to giving in and actually getting help. Yes, you are sick. Yes, you do need HELP! Waiting to get help can lead to far more dangerous results such as extreme blood loss or toxic megacolon.

I spent day after day driving to school and then going to the hospital to stay with my father. I put aside everything in my life to help care for him, and be available for support. My father underwent three extensive surgeries, and with each surgery I suffered relentless worry about the possible complications that could have happened as a result of these surgeries. He was very sick.

At no point in time were we given any information about the Specific Carbohydrate Diet (SCD)™. While we were given a list of foods that were "low fiber" there was no real diet restriction during the entire course of his disease. He no longer battles ulcerative colitis yet does not have his colon.

About one year after my father's battle with ulcerative colitis, Tucker began to have similar symptoms. A huge weight sat on my chest the first time I saw bloody diarrhea in the toilet. I couldn't help but think, "Am I spreading this crap around or what? This cannot be happening!"

I am not implying that one person deserves to have such an awful disease over another, but of all the people in the world, Tucker didn't deserve this. I have never met, or even believed that there could be a person in the universe as kind, generous, trusting, and loving as Tucker. I pinch myself just to make sure that I am actually married to this man. I know it's corny but I love him more and more every day I am with him.

Having said this though, playing the role of caregiver is not all peaches and cream. Your needs have to be set aside, sometimes, for long periods of time in order to take care of your ill loved one. This can be a difficult time in a relationship because you have to be the strong one and the main provider of support.

The emotions you live with when you have a disease such as ulcerative colitis or Crohns are so immense that it requires a great deal of strength, courage, and self-advocacy to maintain a happy and healthy lifestyle. I have cared for people with inflammatory bowel disease in the hospital, in their homes, and within my family, and everyone copes and deals with these diseases in various ways. Most of the patients I care for would never stray from the treatment regimens their doctors put in front of them, yet every day they suffer pain, depression, hopelessness, and ultimately the oh so costly end product of surgery.

As a nurse, I cannot advise patients against a doctor's regimen, and I would never do so, because it would be tremendously unprofessional. So, I go about my nursely duties and hook patients up to parenteral nutrition, which is chock full of sugars, carbs, and all the essential nutrients a person could survive on if they were on a deserted island. All the while I know and say to myself, "I can't believe it is my duty to hook these patients up to "nutrition" which is really making them more sick. I know, and have seen first hand, that the SCD works, and here I am giving this person SUGAR!"

When you go into your doctor's office be prepared for them to not tell you about the SCD, and for the nurses not to advise you on the SCD. The SCD diet manages the symptoms of ulcerative colitis along with a few other diseases, but here is the punch line...It's free! What makes money are the pharmaceutical companies, through all the wonderful medications that are openly and readily prescribed to any and all who come walking through the doors with colitis symptoms. So, the end result is this: SCD is free which equals no money. Prescription medication is expensive which equals more profits, more research, and therefore more prescribing.

Some information is biased and some information is unbiased, so be an educated consumer. Doctors cannot prescribe a diet that does not have the backing of research, but who will fund the research for the SCD when there is no return on investment because it is already free?

One day at work, I was assigned a patient with an admitting diagnosis of "diarrhea". Throughout the day, I repeatedly took this weak patient back and forth to the bathroom, all the while listening to her say things like, "I don't know what this is from," "My doctor said I just ate something bad," and "No, they aren't going to do a colonoscopy because I just have food poisoning." After each bathroom trip, I would look in the toilet and see the coffee ground bloody diarrhea—a classic symptom of ulcerative colitis. I simply couldn't stand it anymore and walked out to the doctor who was standing at the nurse's station and kindly asked if she was planning a colonoscopy to diagnose ulcerative colitis. She simply told me "No, her labs look OK and I think she just ate some bad food."

I could feel my blood pressure rising and again gently said, "I think she has ulcerative colitis. My father and my husband both suffer from the disease and she has the exact same symptoms."

All the while I was playing dumb, because the worst thing you can do as a bedside nurse is to undermine a physician. The physician told me again she was not going to be changing the treatment plan and simply would be providing antibiotics and sending her home.

I went back to the patient's room and found her sitting on the side of the bed, crying, completely hopeless, scared, and confused. I told her about the SCD diet, and how to access the information. She rapidly scribbled the information on a piece of paper and hid it in her purse, as if she knew I could get into trouble if the doctor discovered the advice I had given her. Both the patient and I knew that "food poisoning" doesn't last for weeks and months. She hugged me, and I saw a small glimpse of hope in her face. Later down the road, I received a letter at work, thanking me for my "kind nursing care". I knew she was on the diet.

Ulcerative colitis affects every aspect of patients and family's lives. It is not a glorious disease that people talk about openly and yes, there are glorious diseases that leave cool scars, and epic surgery stories. People with colitis live with fear of unknown consequences, unanswered questions, and endless recommended medication regimens. They also experience solitude, depression, anxiety, and the always looming fear of surgery with the end result of having your colon sewn to your abdomen, openly excreting feces, gas, and watery fluid.

Not only is there a lack of information regarding UC, there is a lack of information that nurses carry with them when treating these patients. I have seen nurses place these patients in isolation and gown up from head to toe, while whispering outside the room, "Yeah, he has ulcerative colitis." This, in itself, shows that people need further education regarding this disease. Let your guard down ladies, it's not contagious, and doing this makes the patient feel more isolated and diseased.

I have read my husband's book front to back and have cried, laughed, and remembered many patients I cared for who would have benefited from the information contained in this book. As you read through it, I hope that you find hope, strength, courage, and the ability to live beyond the disease of ulcerative colitis. It is not what defines you… you define you. Choose to live a normal life, surrounded by supportive people, and don't let the disease stop you from achieving your dreams. As I watch Tucker deal with ulcerative colitis, I often ask myself "how does he stay so strong and never stray from the diet?" I think about my awful chocolate cravings around that super special time of the month and I can tell you it takes determination, strength, and courage.

Living with the SCD as a central part of our culinary lives has, over time, enhanced our relationship, our joy of cooking together, and our knowledge about what we put into our bodies and how it can ultimately affect our health. Take this diet by the horns, do the research, live the lifestyle and I can personally guarantee you that there will be benefits, which will begin to slowly mend a seemingly broken life.

Katie Sweeney

UC Timeline

July 2005:	First symptoms of UC appear then disappear.
July 2006:	Symptoms return and stick around.
September 2006:	Diagnosed with UC by GI doctor. Started Asacol.
October 2006:	Tried blood type diet with limited relief.
November 2006:	Learn about and buy *Breaking the Vicious Cycle* book but do not start the diet.
December 2006:	Started *Specific Carbohydrate Diet* (SCD) with 70% adherence.
January 2007:	Trip to Hawaii. Start Prednisone along with high dose of Asacol.
February 2007:	Return from Hawaii. Begin SCD 100%. Travel East then to Nevada to climb at Red Rocks.
March 2007:	Healthy and medication free. Fully committed to the diet.
April 2007:	Begin carpentry work in Bonners Ferry, ID. Still healthy and medication free.
May 2007:	First flare-up since starting SCD.
June 2007:	Flare-up continues. Re-start Prednisone and start Colazal.
July 2007:	Second flare-up starts.
August 2007:	Climbing trip to the Bugaboos with friends. Re-start Prednisone yet again.
Sept 07-Feb 08:	Multiple flare-ups. Struggle with having confidence in the SCD but slowly making forward progress.
March 2008:	First flare-up without the need for Prednisone. Using only Colazal. Small breakthrough.
April 2008:	Mountain bike trip to Moab, UT with college. Able to get off all medications for second time.

July 2008:	Traveled to the Yucatan with Katie. Still symptom and medication free.
August 2008:	Move to Boise with Katie and our dog Pepper.
July 2009:	Katie and I get married and travel to the British Virgin Islands (BVI's).
September 2009:	Minor flare-up after eating too many "hidden" illegal ingredients while in the BVI's.
September 2010:	Minor flare-up after starting student teaching.
December 2010:	Begin writing this book.

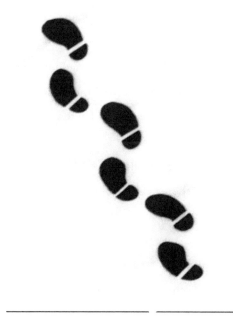

Introduction

~Me, Myself, and UC~

Looking back upon my life before ulcerative colitis (UC), it seems like such a simple time. Most day's, thoughts of medications, food ingredients, and restroom locations were simply absent from my mind. I took these things for granted back then, and used them when I wanted and how I best saw fit. My body was working like it should and I was enjoying all it could give me with little thought of things going wrong. Like most people, I had the beautiful luxury of feeling like major illness would not intrude on my life; like somehow I would be exempt from its cold and firm grasp. I was healthy, young, and able-bodied. What could possibly happen to me?

Most of the time, people who are not sick cannot fully grasp the realities that disease throws at the sufferer. You end up eating, breathing, and thinking about the disease 24/7. Worse yet, as an inflammatory bowel disease (IBD) sufferer you are reminded of your condition multiple times a day as it stares back at you from the toilet. There is no need to seek the confirmation from a doctor that you are sick—you already know it. It whispers to you during the night while you are bleeding, sweating, and cramping on the toilet. It shouts at you when you catch a glimpse of the gaunt figure standing in front of the mirror. And finally, it laughs at you when you are in public, and have to run and hide, seeking refuge within the confines of restroom walls.

Along with many others, I have decided to try and end this nightmare by way of diet and lifestyle modifications, in particular by following the Specific Carbohydrate Diet™ or SCD™. This is a form of healing from the inside out, if you will. Is it hard? Yes. Did the SCD work for me and countless others? Yes. What is holding you back from giving it a shot? Only yourself.

When you or someone you love is diagnosed with an IBD, two questions arise: What is the disease and what can I do about it? Some theories suggest the cause could be pathogenic organisms, an abnormal immune response, or an antigen/bacterial overgrowth. The basic fact is no one really knows the root cause of IBD or how to fully cure it. This leaves the patient and the medical profession with the task of not curing the disease, but managing it.

Since there is no cure for IBD, management choices may include one or more of the following options. The first option usually involves medications like steroids, anti-inflammatory meds, or immune suppressors. This is usually the first thing your doctor will insist you do, and what I chose to do initially. During my experience and meetings with fellow people who suffer from IBD disorders like Crohns disease and ulcerative colitis, there seem to be those who find good results with medication, and others, like myself, who do not. For me, the medications would work for a while and then gradually lose effectiveness, forcing me to seek other options and treatments. Even if you do start the SCD diet, many people find that they need to have the aid of medications to begin the healing process.

The second option people tend to follow is to take the disease and treatment into their own hands, and try to manage, cure or control their condition through diet, supplements or other lifestyle changes. I chose to follow this route and to pursue a better quality of life by following the Specific Carbohydrate Diet. Created by the work of Dr. Sydney Hass and Elaine Gottshall, and later publicized in the book, *Breaking the Vicious Cycle*, Gottshall brings to light the relief that diet modifications can have on disorders such as: Crohns disease, ulcerative colitis, celiac disease, autism, and IBS along with many others. In a nutshell, the theory behind the diet is that by eliminating lactose, grains, sugar, and starchy vegetables (along with other specific foods) you are able to control and manage the bad bacteria that is wreaking havoc on your digestive system; essentially starving that bacteria.

Her book details the science behind the diet, as well as how to get started, and is a must read for anyone considering it. There are also many resources on the Web for "legal/illegal" foods while following the SCD, as well as advice from others who have made the diet a way of life. Yes, the diet is hard to follow, but in my opinion it is nothing compared to living a life with a disease like UC or Crohns. I have talked to many people who have an IBD or know someone who does about my experience. Some give the SCD a try and achieve renewed health. Some give it a try and give up. Others simply can't commit to the lifestyle change that is needed to succeed. In the end it's all up to you.

The last option for many people suffering with IBD is surgery. For those with Crohns, surgery may be a chronic repetitive occurrence that does not necessarily put an end to the symptoms. For those that suffer from uncontrollable UC, surgery may be the only answer to end the symptoms, and for many this option does stop the effect of the disease due to its general isolation in the large intestine or colon. Surgery does, however, come with its fair share of side effects and complications for the majority who elect to have it. For starters, you no longer have your colon to take out all of the water in your stool and you no longer have the storage to hold all of your feces. What does this mean? Well, you end up having to time your meals, and consequently your digestion throughout the day and night in order to be able to pass the waste at appropriate times. This is if you are lucky enough to have a bowel re-section and not end up with a colostomy bag that is attached externally to your colon. This method, though generally effective, can cause not only physical pain but also mental angst and stress. There is also the risk of complications due to pouchitis, which is when the internal or external pouch or surrounding tissue becomes inflamed and needs to have additional surgery or medications to lower the inflammation. All in all surgery should not be taken lightly and is not a quick fix by any stretch of the imagination.

I am not here to tell anyone that one method of treatment is better than the other or that my advice or opinion is superior to anyone else's, especially your doctor's or your own judgment. My goal in writing this book is to share my experience with UC and consequently how I manage it with the SCD diet.

I chose a method of diet modification, such as the SCD for many reasons. First, to me it just makes sense that a disease that is located in your food processing organs has something to do with the food that you are eating! "You are what you eat" was a slogan in my household while growing up and still is to this day.

The food of today is filled with so many substances that neither have a proven track record of safety nor a pronounceable name, much less any practical use. Is it a coincidence that the rates of IBD and other allergies have grown considerably while at the same time the ingestion of processed foods, genetically modified foods, and pesticides have also grown?

I don't claim to have definitive answers to these questions, but I do persuade you to be proactive in knowing where your food comes from and what it is that you are putting into your body. Ask tough questions about your lifestyle and what factors may be contributing to your health situation. Seek advice from the medical profession, but also use common sense and hunt for answers on your own and through people you know. Use a scientific method of gathering information from lots of sources and locations to form your conclusions and plan of action.

The second reason I chose the SCD was because of the amount of support the diet has from people who actually follow it. I was told about the diet from two friends who followed it with huge success, and I continually got the same advice, which was: if you just stick with it, it will work. Use the

Internet to peruse the plethora of websites that either have advice or testimonials of the diets effectiveness. The SCD is something that you yourself have to do. There are no products or potions to buy and no simple pill to take. The diet takes work and means going back to the basics. This means preparing most meals from scratch. It means making food a way of life and nourishment instead of convenience and impulse.

The intention of this book is to provide guidance and support for those who are thinking about starting the SCD, or are currently following it. Other sources provide a wealth of knowledge detailing the science. I have UC and follow the SCD to maintain my health. When I was going through the many ups and downs I encountered I wished I had had a book like this to help guide me.

Lastly, I wouldn't be writing this and I wouldn't be in support of the SCD, if it didn't work for me, but it did. I am in utter awe that I went from being in such poor health and mental exhaustion to living a life of vibrant health and well being. My life now is no longer dictated by restroom locations and distances, no longer filled with uncertainties about remissions and relapses, drugs, cures, and hopeless futures. Instead, I am living life on my terms, not UC terms. I have dreams and aspirations, goals and projects, places to go, and people to see.

It is my opinion that the SCD is not a cure but rather a healthy way to manage the symptoms of UC. Some people may be able to gradually introduce more "illegal" foods after a considerable time on the diet but for many, myself included, this is really not the case. This is why I like the term lifestyle change instead of diet. I changed my lifestyle to suit my new needs of having a disease, and now that I have succeeded and witnessed the change it has brought, I would have it no other way, disease or not. You see the SCD is not just about restricting this food and that food, but rather about trying new foods and ingredients in different combinations. It's about learning to cook chicken soup from scratch and from wholesome ingredients instead of from a can. It's about creating bread from almond flour instead of from wheat flour. People look and act differently from each other so why should our eating habits and health requirements be the same?

I love the way I eat, and I'm grateful for the lessons UC has taught me about health, nutrition, and courage. I implore you to take your own journey of health discovery and find what works for you. Along the way challenge yourself to think beyond the preconceived notions about diet and health and instead focus on what you need now to get better. Be open to the positive and healthy changes this may bring to your life.

Introduction

From a Moms Perspective

My name is Carol Thompson and I am Tucker Sweeney's mom. I am writing as a support person in the life of someone with an IBD. Tucker and I decided to write this book together because the SCD lifestyle is often a team effort, especially in the beginning.

The support person is there to help cook, research, listen, talk to doctors, and to encourage their suffering loved one to keep moving in a forward, positive direction even when things aren't going well. I helped Tucker find appetizing recipes for his new diet and went grocery shopping for him if he was unable to because of a flare-up. I researched doctors, new or alternative treatments, books about the disease, web sites, and communicated with friends who had the disease, all while trying to cheer up his wavering spirit.

We have learned so much along the way and always lamented that there wasn't a more detailed book to help us cope with not only the disease, but also a whole new diet that had to be adhered to 100 percent.

When Tucker wasn't prepared for a certain dietary situation away from home, he suffered. When we were tired of cooking, and he ate eggs and cheese over and over again, he suffered. If we didn't have appetizing foods available, he would lose weight and get into a mental funk. So much was trial and error and more suffering on Tuckers part as we learned more about the disease, the SCD, and the pitfalls to avoid. Is three pieces of fruit too much in one day? What was causing gas and bloating? Are these symptoms normal? Was a relapse while strictly following the diet normal? When do you cry Uncle and take Prednisone and other UC drugs during a relapse? How do other people handle these problems?

We vowed one day to write a book to help people newly diagnosed with this disease or those who wanted to explore a new option of diet if drugs by themselves were no longer working. There are also those, who, just like Tucker, want a higher level of health without the constant addition of medications.

When Tucker decided he was ready to write this book about his experiences living with UC, he asked for my observations of his journey and to add some insight for the support person who may be reading this book. I agreed and realized I had a lot of helpful information to share.

Two Steps Forward, One Step Back

~A Journey Through Life~ Ulcerative Colitis and the Specific Carbohydrate Diet^{TM}

Chapter 1

~Beginnings~

My name is Tucker Sweeney and I have ulcerative colitis. I am twenty-eight years old as I write this, yet the problems within my body started years earlier. Every story has a beginning and an end, and mine begins when I was twenty-three. This is my story.

Like many young men I had dreams, aspirations, and places I wanted to see. I had begun my studies at North Idaho College the previous year and was excited to start classes again. NIC, as everyone calls it, is located in Coeur d' Alene, Idaho, a small city on the lake in the northern portion of the state. I had secured a great job working at the college outdoor program, which happened to be located right on the water in a beach hut during the summers. We rented sea and lake kayaks, sailboats, canoes, and rafts along with selling concessions and other outdoor gear. The environment at the beach hut was outstanding. I started my days by opening up the hut at nine or ten and preparing to do business for the day. Some days the prevailing morning winds turned out to be too good to pass up, forcing me to do my duty and head out on one of the catamarans to "test" the lake conditions. Simply said life was good.

I have always been a healthy person. I exercised frequently and ate a healthy, well-rounded diet. I was rarely sick, had no food or environmental allergies, and had limited exposure to chemicals and antibiotics. It was a rare occasion when I suffered from diarrhea and had no family history of colitis, Crohns, or other bowel disorders. I took care of my body, and under most circumstances, it took care of me.

The previous July, I was sick with symptoms of stomach pain, explosive diarrhea, and gas. When it didn't go away after a couple of weeks, I went into one of the health clinics in the area and had a battery of tests done:

blood workup, stool culture, physical exam, etc. with nothing found. The

closest thing the doctors could align my symptoms with was that I had contracted a bacterium like Giardia from drinking from an untreated water source; something I had done a few times while on hikes in the backcountry

 Fact Check

The Crohns & Colitis Foundation of America estimates that there are 1.4 million Americans that have an IBD.[4]

mountains. I was told to wait another week and if the symptoms persisted I would need to return and get on an antibiotic or some other antibacterial medication to stop the unknown invader in my body. About a week later my symptoms suddenly stopped and before long I had forgotten all about the mysterious three-week sickness I had endured.

For the rest of the year, I remained healthy and continued to go to school with a newly chosen major in K-12 physical education. My cousin Andrew and I bought a house in downtown Coeur d' Alene and were enjoying life as homeowners/real estate investors, as we liked to think of ourselves. Our house was conveniently located near the many downtown bars. The weekend ritual was to head out of the house filled with excitement and liquid courage, then wander back to the house confused, tired and queasy. This seemed the natural thing for a twenty something to do, or so I thought.

Besides the normal scene of college and home life, I was deeply entrenched in the sport of rock climbing and would pine for hours over the various guidebooks that littered my room. I had first been exposed to the sport at age twelve by my dad Joe and my uncle Kevin. I can still remember the knee knocking fear that I experienced at the top of my first rappel. I was not able to commit to lowering myself off the edge and was instead frozen at the lip with a death grip on the brake hand; therefore not moving up or down, just stuck. Soon enough though you make a choice to go with it or

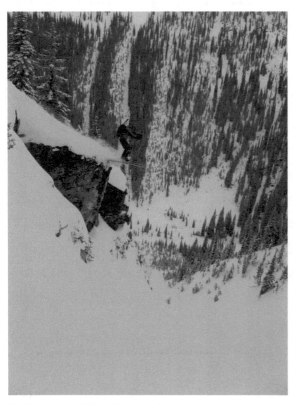

Backcountry skiing in Canada

give up and go home. I knew I was at the brink of something very exciting; something that I felt could carry me on a very stimulating journey. I made that step, and as my white knuckled fingers loosened and allowed the rope to pass through my hands, I slowly started to descend. At this point I knew I was on to something great.

At age fifteen I met Kale and Winter, who would become my closest friends at a local, newly exposed climbing area. Yes I know, just about the most common names in the book, right? That day we met up and climbed until dark on what we would later find out was private property and dirty, grungy rock. To us though, it didn't matter because we had found something that was exciting, different, and dangerous. With those key ingredients we would form a strong partnership and friendship, in which we trusted each other's lives and pushed one another to exceed our personal limits.

During the year after my mysterious illness, Kale, Winter, and I managed to climb throughout the Western states. We climbed everything we could get our hands on, from 500 foot desert towers in Utah to routes in the valleys of rural Idaho, to thousand foot granite spires in British Columbia. In the wintertime we would backcountry ski into the snowy landscapes of the nearby mountains of Canada, as well as explore the ski terrain near my hometown of Bonners Ferry, Idaho. The thrill of carving tracks into snow that was untouched and hard to access excited us and encouraged the pursuit of earning our turns the hard way; sans chairlift or snow cat.

As spring approached I was nearing the end of my second year at NIC and was looking forward to the summer season and my newly acquired job at the Outdoor Pursuits beach hut. Until that time no thought of the strange GI problems I encountered the previous year crossed my mind. I thought it was simply a strange bug I had picked up, and was now rid of. This was, however, going to change and end up altering my life and lifestyle altogether.

 Fact Check

An article about the SCD diet that was featured in The Crohns & Colitis Foundation of America website remarks that, "Studies are expensive and someone has to pay," Dr. Loftus says. "Most clinical studies in this country are funded by pharmaceutical companies, he notes, and since there's no potential drug at stake with this diet, it would be difficult to find the funding".[6]

It's Not The Flu

Tucker has just emailed me the introduction he wrote for this book. As I read it my stomach clenches, the tears flow, and I am transported back to a mother's worst nightmare.

It all started with a phone call from Tucker. I could hear the stress in his voice as he described the awful flu symptoms he had dealt with for over a week—intense cramping with diarrhea all day, which was starting to interrupt his sleep at night.

He was living about 100 miles south of us where he owned a home and attended college. He had finished final exams a couple months prior and had thought the initial symptoms were just related to the rigors of testing. The same symptoms had appeared last year around the same time. They had stuck around for a few weeks and just when we were getting concerned, they mysteriously disappeared.

I convinced Tucker to come home for a few days while he recovered and I would make him some homemade chicken noodle soup. I was especially concerned when he said he was losing a lot of weight. I wanted him to see our family practitioner while he was here. I also hoped I wouldn't get this flu bug too; it seemed like a particularly nasty one.

As the mother of two active adventurous sons, I carry my share of worries about them but I remember not being too concerned until I saw Tucker get out of his car a couple hours later. As he stood up in our driveway I felt a wave of shock run through me. His clothes hung on his medium frame and his face was gaunt; eyes sunken in their sockets. Worse, he was stooped over, walking like an old man. No trace of my vibrant, active twenty-three year old son. What kind of a flu bug was this? Where was my adrenaline junkie son who loved climbing up 1000-foot cliffs every weekend?

I put a smile on my face as I approached him but worry was already starting to cloud my mind. I think I knew then that something was seriously wrong but it was easy to deny as Tucker had always been so healthy and strong, never sick, even as a child. I could only remember him going to the doctor a couple times in his childhood due to illness. Broken bones and injuries of active boys were why we went to the doctors while sickness rarely struck our household.

Our hugs were quick as he hurried into the house towards the bathroom, but I'd still had a chance to feel the bones in his normally muscular back through his shirt. The hair on the back of my neck prickled, but I still had no idea of the challenges that lay ahead for my son. I still thought it was the flu.

I quickly asked if there was any blood in his stool and he replied he hadn't seen any and then the bathroom door slammed shut. Thank God I thought, relief flooding my body. But just as quickly, my mind raced back to a day when he was four years old and we were playing the game called Candyland. Tucker had drawn a green card then moved his piece to a red square. "You need to put your man on the same color square as the card you just drew" I instructed. "I did!" Tucker shouted. "Does that color look green to you?" I asked as we both looked at the red square. I was holding the green card next to the red square for emphasis. "Yes!" he yelled "THEY ARE THE SAME COLOR!" I knew then that Tucker was colorblind.

"I better check for myself to see if there is any blood", I recall saying to Tucker through the closed bathroom door. "Remember, you are colorblind and may not be able to distinguish if there is any blood in the toilet bowl." He consented in between spasms of cramping and diarrhea. After several minutes he emerged from the bathroom hunched over and shaking with weakness. I helped him to the guest bed so he could lie down then went back to inspect the toilet bowl for any signs of blood. What I saw in the bathroom made my knees buckle under me. This was no flu bug and something was seriously wrong with my son. The toilet bowl was filled with bright red blood.

 Fact Check

The results of Dr. Leo Galland's study of the SCD: "...*All 20 patients demonstrated a decrease in symptoms and reduction in medication use. Six patients have entered complete clinical remission, discontinued all medication, and maintained in remission for five to 80 months...*".[7]

Chapter 2

~A Change for the Worse~

July 12th, it was mid-season at the beach hut and things were going smoothly. The weather was nice and hot and sales at the hut had been steadily rising. I tried to take any chance I could to get onto the water in a catamaran or sunfish to hone my skills. Stormy weather was now my favorite time to go out on the water. It gave me a thrill unlike anything else I had done thus far. Skimming along the water with a perfect tack holding my sails and caressing the water with my extended fingers brought a great feeling of freedom and contentment.

Around the 20th of July, I started noticing that I had to visit the restroom more often than usual, and the urgency of these visits was starting to increase. As this book is about UC I think most people reading this will know that when I refer to having to go to the restroom it was not to urinate but rather for a bowel movement or BM. I can easily remember these trips to the restroom because at the time the beach hut had no real bathroom on the premises. Instead, I had to take a couple minute's walk, or in my case a 30 second run, to a nearby set of port-a-potties that were on another section of the beach.

I noticed that my BM's began to contain lots of mucus and water and left me feeling drained and fatigued, especially in a 100-degree port-a-potty! After about two weeks I had absolutely no formed BM's and all were accompanied by a fierce urgency that gave me a look of "get the hell out of the way!" while running to the restroom. As for other symptoms, I had plenty of mind-bending gas that made me wish for the sound of a full throttle chainsaw to give me privacy while doing my business. Trust me, if you have UC or Crohns and are reading this, you know what I mean. I also started to get really intense abdominal cramps, both in my entire abdominal area and localized on my descending colon (left side). The cramps were so bad that I would have to start breathing like I was in labor or something and they would usually last for two to five minutes. After three weeks of this I knew something was not right and that whatever I had come down with a year ago was back, and with teeth this time. I called my mom and she convinced me to come to her house to rest. While there, she discovered blood in my stool that my color blindness had prevented me from detecting, and she immediately contacted her doctor.

Hoping it was Giardia, the doctor prescribed me the anti-bacterial medication Flagyl, and warned me not to drink any alcohol. Flagyl was previously used as a punishment therapy for alcoholics because of the extreme nausea it causes when alcohol and Flagyl come in contact with each other. So, for the next two weeks I went on the wagon, but failed to see any change in my condition. At this point I was really starting to lose weight and my face was beginning to become gaunt and pale. I was now passing only liquid, which left the toilet water dark with what looked to be blood. My mind began to spin with the notion that something was seriously wrong.

On day ten, I went to a clinic in Coeur d' Alene to find out what theory they would enlighten me with next. The doctor there thought I might have a large bleeding internal hemorrhoid and with my consent decided to take an immediate look. Let me tell you, this was neither glamorous nor manly. Before I knew it, the doctor and her young, cute female assistant had my ankles in stirrups above my head and a clear plastic probe you know where. After beaming a light up where the sun-don't-shine, they confirmed that the entire lining of my rectum was badly inflamed and covered in blood and mucus. After this discovery I was quickly referred to a gastroenterologist (G.I.) doctor in town and given the number to call to make an appointment.

Previous to my up and coming diagnosis of UC, I had never even heard of inflammatory bowel diseases like UC or Crohns. As far as I knew the only things you had to look out for with your digestive system were certain kinds of cancers. As fate would have it though, several months before my diagnosis I found out what a disease like UC had to offer.

I had begun to date a girl named Katie and it just so happened that her dad had UC. The first time I met him; Katie and I drove an hour north to his house. He needed help doing some things around the house because he was too sick to move from the couch. At this point I had no idea what UC was, what the symptoms were or what it could do to you.

When we arrived at his house the tiny man that lay on the couch shocked me. He had to whisper his words due to fatigue and pain and had gone from 160lb to 115lb in a matter of months. The man that lay in front of me, in my opinion, looked more like an AIDS patient than someone suffering from an ulcerating colon. Katie and I proceeded to gather some groceries together for him including a couple gallons of whole milk in the hopes he could put on some weight. I mowed his lawn, and even though he could hardly talk, he managed to lecture me about the right and wrong way to mow a lawn and how not to kill his quirky lawn mower, which I promptly proceeded to kill, and in turn received a "told you so" moment.

Two weeks later, Katie's Dad had to have an emergency large intestine removal due to the lining of his colon literally disintegrating from all of the ulceration and inflammation.

The meeting with Katie's dad was my first interaction with an IBD disease. Though I still knew very little about it I saw it could be very serious and debilitating. I left her dad's house after that first meeting, glad to have lent a hand, yet sorry about the health problems he had to endure. I would soon confront this condition for myself, and have the tables turned so that I was the one that needed help, not the one giving it.

Chapter 3

~The Nightmare Unfolds~

Life at the beautiful beach hut and at home gradually became a worsening nightmare. I was now concerned with only two things—when the next urgent attack would hit, and how close I was to the nearest toilet. At this point I had been referred to a G.I. doctor after my bloody examination at the clinic earlier. The problem though, was that my appointment was a month away. When I calmly explained to the receptionist that my condition could not wait an entire month, she calmly replied that, "if it's an emergency or you can't wait, then you need to go to the emergency room and be admitted there." Having an immediate admittance did sound really tempting but the extremely high cost of a visit did not sit well with my poverty level college bank account. So, what did my cheap ass do? I waited, and I waited.

Waiting a month while having something horrific like UC tear through your body was not an easy thing to do. The doctor at the clinic obviously knew something serious was going on with me but he could only pass me on to the next doctor. Why was it so difficult to find answers and help for my worsening condition and why won't anyone seem to help me?

Katie was obviously fearful after recently watching her father almost die from his ulcerated colon literally falling apart inside his body and just barely escaping the hands of death. We stay hooked to the phone, calling anyone who might have advice on how to get anyone in the healthcare profession to help. But of course, there just simply was no G.I. doctor willing to see me. It was almost like having someone say, "Just wait and see if you bleed to death, until we can work you into the doctors schedule."

At this point I was having a BM about 15-20 times in a 24-hour period. The mornings and nights were especially tiring and I learned to survive on very little sleep. I started to also experience side effects of UC like joint pain, which I felt in my lower back and hips. During the night I would have to lie on my back with a pillow under my knees and try to not move. Trying not to move only lasts so long when you have to get up every hour and hobble to the toilet all through the night. If I tried to sleep on my side, which was my preferred way to sleep, it would immediately cause me to have a BM. I believe that lying on your side, especially your left side, which contains your descending colon, can cause you to have a BM because your colon is more relaxed in this position.

During the day, I had the least symptoms but early mornings were the worst. Mornings were like a hot day in hell. The moment I cracked an eye I immediately needed to go to the bathroom, even if I felt no urge to do so. Morning time was the cleanout time for my colon, but unlike people with normal intestines mine was not something you look forward to. No, morning time for me was more similar to having labor contractions with bloody diarrhea while at the same time feeling like I had to vomit. Plus, the waves of squeezing peristalsis that move things along your digestive tract were way out of sync. I would be sitting on the toilet thinking I'm done, so I would begin to stand up, only to immediately have to sit down again as another wave hit. Up down, up down, up down, until finally my colon would stop contracting and I could leave the bathroom.

I had also become a public bathroom connoisseur. Upon entering a new building or store I would quickly have the bathrooms scoped out and try to gain a feeling of how busy they were. My town of Coeur d' Alene had become a maze of bathroom locations. I knew which were the clean ones, how busy they were, if they were noisy enough, and if the locks worked. I had my favorite spots located around campus, usually some small bathroom on a forgotten floor that would reward me with a certain degree of privacy. I was no longer amongst the normal people while out and about. Instead I was living my life surrounded by tile, porcelain, and if I was lucky, a locked door.

I would sit there, head in my hands, face perspiring from the intense contractions, all the while trying to not slip down the spiraling path of depression and anxiety. These were very lonely times; times of learned helplessness, which invaded my thoughts and robbed me of the pleasures in life. Was this some kind of sick joke or punishment God was throwing at me? What had I done to deserve this? UC is not a disease that friends and family send get well cards for, rather it is something few understand or want to understand. Hell, it's hard to even explain to your closest friends, let alone a new acquaintance, " Hi, my name is Tucker Sweeney and I have 15-20 explosive bowel movements a day, what was your name again?"

Dating or even thinking about dating is a whole other cluster as well. How are you supposed to explain to your new date that most likely during dinner or a movie you will need to rush off multiple times for no reason? Blaming it on the water only gives you a couple of passes and before long you will need to come clean. But how? "Oh by the way, I have a bowel disease that causes me to visit the crapper every hour. More popcorn?"

The facts of life with UC require that you know someone at a certain level, that you are comfortable with them, and they with you. The problem though, is that UC is hard to keep hidden from those around you. It finds you at work, it accompanies you when you exercise, and it even fills your senses when you are building a romantic relationship. Anxiety over these matters can start to infiltrate many of your day-to-day functions and can even make your condition worse. Rather than simply thinking about regular day-to-day activities, I now had relentless fears like, how am I going to take a two-hour exam without leaving in the middle to go to the bathroom? Of course the professor always says something along the lines of, "you cannot leave the testing room, until you are completely done or else you will not have a passing grade." Fail or crap my pants? Hmmm, big decision. For some, this anxiety becomes too much, and consequently they start restricting their outings and shying away from personal interactions. Besides, it wasn't much fun going out anyway when all I could think about was when I would have a BM, where it would take place, and if I could get there quick enough.

In order to still maintain a job during the day and prepare myself for the upcoming schedule of college classes, I started to modify my eating habits to suit my digestive timetable. I no longer ate breakfast, so that the last food I had eaten the previous evening was totally gone from my system. My first meal tended to be around 1:00pm, which was really hard at first but soon became routine. I generally found that I tended to lose about the same amount of weight by not eating as I did from eating and then having ravaging diarrhea. Either way, the weight was coming off at alarming speed and at this point I looked strikingly thin and gaunt. My neck was thinning out making my head look like a ball of cotton candy on its stick. The skin around my face became increasingly thin, causing my cheekbones to protrude and my eyes to look sunken within their sockets. I needed help and I needed it soon.

Chapter 4

~The Diagnosis~

My day at the doctors finally came and I had my mom come down to accompany me to the office. We sat in the waiting room for what seemed like an eternity, along with other patients, most of whom were elderly. Finally, a middle-aged doctor came through one of the large wooden doors and called my name. We went into one of the exam rooms and he proceeded to ask questions about my symptoms, family history, etc. After about 15 minutes of this he said that it sounded to him like a classic case of UC but that the only true way to find out was to have a colonoscopy or a sigmoidoscopy.

A couple of minutes later he said, "Well, if you want to find out right now we can do the limited sigmoidoscopy downstairs in the clinic?"

I thought about it for a second, remembering my last fun adventure with the stirrups and lights but decided to go for it. I was whisked downstairs to the lab and procedure floor and ushered into a room with a large TV on one wall. From there I was instructed to get into a butt-less gown and lay down on the examination table. The doctor and his assistant soon entered the room and I was told to roll onto my left side then relax and watch. Before I knew it the lube was out, and up with the periscope they went, all of it in high definition no less.

Most people who get a full colonoscopy are put out for the procedure and now I know why. To keep your colon large and away from the scope they continually blow air into it to make it inflate and provide a large passageway. This continual air pressure going up and down was not very comfortable and made me feel like I had to take a BM at every turn. The doctor and I traveled up through my colon and at almost every turn we witnessed the destruction of UC. There would be patches of healthy pink tissue then patches of dark, red tissue that oozed blood and mucus. The farther we went the more of a sinking feeling I began to have. This was not something that would be a quick fix, and the visions of Katie's sick dad on the couch continued to storm through my thoughts. When the doctor had seen enough and had taken multiple biopsies of colon tissue, he reversed course and the procedure came to a close.

Later in the week, I had a follow-up visit with the same GI doctor. He quickly informed me that I did indeed have UC and that the disease was at a moderate phase of inflammation. I remember sitting there in shock with an overwhelming feeling of anxiety over my condition. Would this be something that would never go away? Would I have to live my life like this day in, and day out?

I was prescribed Asacol and informed that most people respond very well to this type of medication, many being able to return to a normal life. Would this be me? Would I be able to return to the life I had previously known? One not dictated by restroom locations and digestion timetables? Even though I was not thrilled about being tied to expensive drugs the thought of gaining relief sounded like a dream.

 Fact Check

The net sales of Asacol were $660 million dollars in 2010. Of this $660 million, $589 million of revenues came from the United States alone.[1]

The Doctors Visit

We were sitting in the gastroenterologist's office waiting to see the doctor. Tucker was trying to find a comfortable way to sit in his chair. Waiting a month for an appointment had taken its toll on his now frail body. Diarrhea and cramping were his constant companions. I was there to help him deal with a diagnosis that we knew wasn't going to be pretty. We had been using the Internet to look up symptoms of weight loss plus cramping with bloody diarrhea, and the words Crohns and ulcerative colitis kept flashing on the screen. We were saddened over the prospect of a life altering diagnosis, but at the same time anxious to understand and treat what was happening to his body. I needed to know the enemy that was attacking my son's health so, as a mother, I could fight back.

The helpless feeling of waiting for an appointment one month away while watching Tuckers body disintegrate had been heartbreaking for me. We were told to go to the emergency room if he couldn't wait for an appointment but that would cost a minimum of one thousand dollars just to be admitted. Tucker didn't have insurance and insisted he could hang on for four more weeks. Those long thirty days were filled with worry and stress for me, sleepless nights with endless diarrhea and cramping for Tucker. I remember taking showers and quietly letting the tears flow as the warm water washed over my face. I prayed constantly for God to switch the disease to my body. My twenty-three year old son was just starting his life. Please God, let him live a normal life became my constant thought. I called other doctor's offices but they couldn't get him in any sooner. I found myself becoming transfixed on the mission at hand, and angry about the difficult process of seeking medical help. Tucker looked as if he would be about dead by the time his GI appointment came around!

Now, a month later, we were anxiously awaiting our turn to see the GI specialist; me, lost in my thoughts of my sons future and Tucker getting up to go to the bathroom every fifteen minutes as the anxiety of the moment took hold of his guts and squeezed. Suddenly it was our turn and we followed the nurse to the examination room. I listened as Tucker told his symptoms to the doctor who nodded his head as if already knowing the answer. It sounds like UC, he told us but to be absolutely sure we need to do a biopsy, and whisked my son off to his surgical room to perform a sigmoidoscopy. I anxiously awaited the news, which was a confident "yes" that Tucker's colon looked like a classic case of ulcerative colitis and the biopsy would later confirm this. We were sent home with a prescription for medication and the doctor's parting words that diet and stress don't matter. Eat what you want, do what you want; the medicine will help get your symptoms under control.

The web sites we browsed daily also took this approach of just sit back and let the medicine do its thing. If that particular medicine doesn't work then try another more potent one. The Asacol was a miraculous lifeline and did indeed get Tucker's symptoms under control. Within three days he was feeling better and getting some much needed sleep at night. We were grateful for the quick relief of symptoms, however, we didn't know what 'under control' meant, and the possible side effects were scary to read about. I decided to do some research myself as Tucker was still resting and regaining his strength.

I contacted a friend of ours who had moved to Washington State. Don had battled UC when he and his family were our close neighbors years ago. I was introduced to the words ulcerative colitis after witnessing Don fight this mysterious disease and grow deathly ill. It was a long recovery for him but I had heard he now exuded excellent health. I seemed to remember a diet being the reason for his many years of well-being, and wanted to talk to him about it. Tucker, however, wasn't ready to talk on the phone to another man about the horrors of diarrhea and living with UC so it was up to me to make the call.

It was reassuring talking to Don and he told me to immediately get my hands on the book, *Breaking The Vicious Cycle* and have Tucker follow the diet one hundred percent. Don also warned me there was a lot of cooking involved with the SCD diet and Tucker would need assistance preparing food and planning meals while he adjusted to his new way of life. Anything would be easier than watching my son spiral down into the pits of hell with this disease so I rolled up my sleeves and prepared myself to start cooking! Besides, I really did enjoy cooking, and was fairly skilled at it. I felt some relief talking to Don as I embraced the much-needed advice from someone who'd walked in Tucker's shoes already. I felt like we were finally getting some answers.

Don ended our conversation by saying that his diagnosis of UC introduced him to eating an incredibly healthy diet using SCD guidelines, and for that he was extremely grateful. He was much healthier now than he had ever been in his life. My mind couldn't quite wrap around the idea of Tucker being healthier after a diagnosis of UC but I trusted Don's enthusiasm for the changes in his life and health that the SCD diet had blessed him with. He also warned me that Tucker needed to commit to this new lifestyle for himself and he may have to hit rock bottom before he was ready to make the changes needed to follow such a restrictive diet. The tightness in my shoulders was easing, and the lump in my throat was getting smaller. I still cried in the shower from the sheer terror of all we'd gone through, and for the challenges that lay ahead. We felt like we were walking blind into unknown territory but at least we were developing a support group of people to help guide us when we were feeling lost and scared.

I was ready to tackle this new diet for Tucker but my son didn't quite want to follow the SCD one hundred percent. He was feeling better on the meds and wanted to explore other options that weren't quite so drastic. On the SCD, no sugar, starches (he lived on sushi, burritos and brewers yeast toast), soy products or chocolate were allowed plus he had to make his own yogurt and eat 2-3 cups of it a day! These were restrictions he wasn't ready to commit to just yet.

Chapter 5

~Diets, Meds, and Defiance~

Immediately after my doctor visit I headed to the store and bought my very first bottle of prescription Asacol. The first shocker was the $300.00 plus price tag for about a months supply. The second shocker was that I would need to take two pills, three times a day, for an indefinite amount of time. Six pills a day? To me, this seemed like a lot. I didn't even like taking a multi-vitamin and preferred to rely on eating well, only taking vitamins on an "as needed" basis.

After 3-4 days on the meds I started to feel a gradual easing of symptoms. The frequency of BM's during the night started to lessen, and I was able to introduce more food during the day. One month on Asacol and I was almost back to a normal lifestyle and was no longer held hostage to restroom runs. I felt immense thankfulness to the medication and the doctor for prescribing it, both then and now, but in spite of my relief, I knew deep down that Asacol was not curing the root of the problem but instead just masking it's symptoms. After being on the meds for around 2-3 months the majority of my UC symptoms had gone away.

I began to look for alternative options to manage or cure my newly diagnosed disease. I talked to friends, went to alternative medicine clinics, and researched information through books and the Internet. Two interesting options appeared to peak my interest: *The Blood Type Diet*™ and the *Specific Carbohydrate Diet* that my moms friend Don was following. I first learned about the *Blood Type Diet* after I went to my local naturopath and explained my situation. We tested my blood and learned that I was type A. According to the diets author, Peter D' Adamo, type A's should eat more grains, tofu, and general carbohydrates instead of meats, fats, and other proteins. I already ate a lot of grains and carbs because they were a cheaper food source on my student budget so this diet didn't seem too drastic. I was excited about trying a new diet for my disease and was confident in its potential positive effects, even though my GI doctor told me plain and simple. " Diet has nothing to do with this disease, don't worry about anything you eat, it just doesn't matter." Really, I remember thinking. Really?

I began following the *Eat Right for Your Blood Type* diet faithfully and it seemed to have some encouraging results. I felt good and my health continued to improve. I was still on Asacol but felt like many do, that my improvements were linked more to my new way of eating than the medications I had started previously. Things went well for about another month until the good old symptoms of UC started creeping back. A little more gas than usual, looser stools, flecks of tissue in the toilet, side pain, etc.

Everyone close to you will try to think on the bright side and say things like, "Don't worry about it, everybody gets an upset stomach or some diarrhea at times," or "Its most likely something you ate, you know my stomach feels a little off too," or the classic one of, "Just stop thinking about it so much, it will pass soon." Only a person with an IBD knows that 9 out of 10 times things will not just "get better". Instead they will progress into agony, anger, and embarrassment. This constant worry and daily "duty" of seeing if things were right or not is one of the worst parts of this disease. The good periods relapsing into bad periods weighs heavily on you as an individual. Its like having heart disease or cancer that comes and goes each month, except that IBD diseases are not glorified or looked upon as heartbreaking, rather they are just something you deal with in private and don't talk about.

Time went by and my disease intensified to at, or beyond, its previous levels, and I settled into the rhythm of living with UC again. I made another visit to the naturopath to discuss my current condition but was met with frustration when he offered me no new tips or options, and instead said,

"Just stick with the plan". Months went by and I "just stuck to the plan", eating lots of tofu, miso, rice, all vegetables, sugar, yet no wheat. I started attending yoga classes and doing meditation exercises at home. My condition had worsened, but I was getting used to dealing with it. I was adjusting to the lack of sleep, and becoming better at timing my meals around my daily errands and obligations, however, I was becoming frustrated at the restrictions the disease caused.

In defiance of my condition I planned a trip to Hawaii with Katie. Katie didn't think I was well enough to take such an extended trip but I insisted. The plan was to go to Kona, on the Big Island, for Katie's sister's wedding, and from there head to Kauai. We had bought one-way tickets and were planning to live on the island for several months. I knew a family friend who lived in Kauai and he had construction work available, which would pay enough to support both of us. We also found an organic farm that offered room and board in exchange for labor on the farm. The idea of taking a semester off to live on a tropical island sounded great and we both counted down the days until we left.

January finally came and the days until take-off grew closer. At this point I had just experienced a three-week remission period in Coeur d' Alene, but with five days until the trip I started to feel the effects of yet another relapse on the horizon. I started to freak out about the fact that I would be stuck sharing a small hotel room with Katie, her mom, and her two sisters with only one bathroom. My head began to spin with anxiety. The sounds that come out during a bathroom adventure with UC can be embarrassing when you are by yourself, let alone while in a small room with others.

This would be my third or fourth flare up since being on Asacol and the *Blood Type Diet* and I figured this would be a good time to try something different. I ended up calling the family friend who had originally talked to my mom about the SCD diet. His name was Don and he too had UC, yet had been symptom free for over eight years while following the diet. I made the call to get the lowdown on the diet and to hear from a friend about the best way to start. The talk with Don was a great experience that to this day I still remember very clearly. We talked about the disease itself, the SCD, and shared stories that only IBD sufferers could relate to, and even laugh about. After talking with Don I decided to re-read *Breaking the Vicious Cycle* (BTVC) and this time paid close attention to the legal/illegal list of foods. I went through my kitchen cabinets and discarded all of the rice, flour, and sugary foods. This cleaning out felt good and is a must do for anyone serious about making a switch to the SCD.

The first major mistake I made, however, was this: I decided that some was better than none and went into the diet with about 70% adherence. I had decided that I would buy unsweetened yogurt from the store instead of making my own 24-hour yogurt. I would eat the occasional sprouted bread from the health food store, and I would not worry about many of the small ingredients that were in many of the foods I consumed. Did I do this because I was ignorant about the phrases "fanatical adherence" or "only works if followed 100%" from the BTVC book? No, not really. Instead I wanted a quick fix in which I could just dip my toe into the cold water, instead of taking the full body plunge. I also didn't commit 100% because I felt that I was already too overwhelmed with the disease and didn't want to give any more time to the whole process. Lastly, I think subconsciously I didn't want to experience another failure in the fight against my illness. The Blood Type Diet wasn't helping, the Asacol had stopped preventing flare-ups, and I was coming closer and closer to the realization that I just might have to either live with this disease in its current state of misery or have surgery; the latter having serious, irreversible unknowns.

Within a couple of days, Katie and I were on our way to the Big Island to meet up with her family and to attend her sisters wedding. I packed nothing special for my diet except the legal/illegal list of foods from BTVC and the phone number of my doctor back home. Thinking back on this moment I feel that I was incredibly brave, yet also naïve about the voyage I was about to take.

After sitting through multiple flights, casting nervous glances towards the bathroom occupied light, we finally touched down at the small open-air airport in Kona. I had been to Kona four years earlier while visiting my Dad, who had been on an extended trip to the island. I had fond memories of the beautiful beaches, some of which were completely black sand, and the wonderful temperatures that rarely moved up or down from eighty degrees. In one word: perfect.

We exited the plane and walked toward the shade of the small terminal. Katie's mom, Anna, who had arrived the day before, greeted us as we grabbed our bags from the small oval baggage claim in the center of the terminal. After saying our alohas we jumped into the rental car and were whisked away to our hotel, which lay on the southern end of the island. Within hours of being at the hotel I knew I needed to go to the store to gather food for my newly acquired diet regimen. At the store I bought a large block of pepper jack cheese, a large quart of unsweetened yogurt, a can of peanuts, bananas, and a pineapple. Back at the hotel, I began to nibble on these foods but soon realized that it was hard to feel full while just snacking. During dinners I tried to choose legal entrees like fish, and other seafood, along with salads. However, when things did not come prepared as I had hoped such as having an unknown sauce over the fish, I chose to eat it instead of complain and send it back. I felt like this was my problem and that it was something I should just keep to myself. At this point, I was also not very knowledgeable about the diet myself and didn't want to bring up random questions to which I did not know the answers.

Committing to the dietary restrictions was made much harder due to the fact that I wasn't seeing any improvement in my condition; in fact, a new and extremely painful flare up was beginning. After a few nights of not sleeping and having to get up throughout the night to use the restroom with four women lying mere feet from the bathroom walls, I had had enough. I was trying all sorts of tricks to mask the sounds that erupted from within the bathroom but none of them really did the trick: turning the faucet on, turning the shower on, flushing the toilet, coughing. Three days after we arrived I made a call to my doctor back home who knew I would be traveling to Hawaii. I explained that I was no longer responding to the Asacol and that my symptoms were intensifying. He wrote me a prescription for Prednisone and an increase of the Asacol from six pills a day to nine. I was not happy about the addition of more pills but I was excited to try something that might afford some relief. I went to a Wal-Mart in town where my Idaho doctor had faxed my prescription. The first shocker of the day was the price of the Prednisone. I was used to paying the astronomical price of Asacol so it was a surprise when the lady asked for a payment of five dollars for a month's supply. Five bucks! Are you kidding me? I thought. Once back at the hotel, like a heroin addict, I quickly went about unwrapping my drug package and reading the labels for dosing information.

The taste of Prednisone is not something you try and remember but rather a taste and sensation you cannot forget. The pills are extremely bitter and their consistency is chalk like, making it hard for them to not get stuck on your tongue or throat while swallowing, thereby prolonging the bitter, burning sensation.

I realized that I was starting to resent the medication that I was now required to take and was becoming angry at the lack of progress I was making, or rather not making, while putting out so much effort. I remembered one of the points that Don had made during our conversation weeks ago. He told me that I had to look at all the therapies I was trying with an equal, positive outlook. Look at the medications as something good and which are helping, not as something I have to do with negative side effects. Doing this would help put my mind at ease and focus all my energy on trying to get better instead

 Fact Check

WebMD reports that Prednisone has 78 known side effects. Some of which include: Bleeding of the Stomach or Intestines, Cataracts, Osteoporosis, Diabetes, Infection, and Hallucination.[5]

of feeling depressed and angry, which accomplished nothing and could have detrimental effects on my health. So, with those thoughts in mind, I took my first dose of Prednisone and hoped for the best.

I was told by Katie's mom, who was a nurse, that the effects of Prednisone usually took between 2-4 days to be felt, and for me this was the case. By the third day, I was visiting the bathroom fewer times during the day and night, yet was a long way from being in the normal range. My hunger was so intense throughout the day that I made the choice, against my better judgment to buy some regular bread and a jar of peanut butter to satisfy my cravings. I would get overwhelmed in the grocery store with all of the choices, almost all of them being things I could not have. I began to hate the fact that I had to buy the same foods over and over again, and would snap at Katie when I threw an item in the cart that she told me had some random illegal ingredient in it. "Don't worry about it!" I would say, trying to remain calm and collected amongst the other shoppers.

The day before the wedding, Katie's sister and her husband-to-be hosted a luau at one of the nearby resorts. The luau was open to the public but still managed to remain small and intimate. There was a huge spread of food, much of which I could legally eat, including grilled fish, ceviche, and traditional roasted/buried pork. The atmosphere was great, the food excellent, and my condition poor. For some reason, even having been on

40mg of Prednisone and nine pills of Asacol a day for multiple days I was not feeling any better during this evening. I would try and carry on conversations with the other guests while at the table but would continually have to excuse myself to use the restroom. Now, as I've written before, I am a bathroom connoisseur and this one I didn't like. It was a dark, dirty little restroom with three urinals and one toilet that had a door that didn't lock. Seeing as this was the only bathroom for a luau that hosted two to three hundred people there was almost always a waiting line. Sometimes I would get lucky and be able to just walk in, and other times I would have to stand in line and just breathe and maintain complete concentration on getting in on time. For some reason this evening was extra tough and I began to feel really ill. I was sweaty and pale and the button up shirt I wore literally hung from my body. My mental capacity at this point was almost completely exhausted. Here I was, in my early twenties; on a beautiful tropical island and all I can think about is this extraordinary cramping in my gut and waves of nausea that poured over my sweating body. No, this is not how I had planned to live my life, and it was certainly not something I felt I deserved. Why me? Why now, in the prime of my life and here on an exotic island with a beautiful girlfriend?

By the end of the evening I had stopped returning to the table and instead had reserved a spot outside the restrooms due to the repeated trips I was taking. I was no longer passing food matter but instead just pure water and blood followed by uncontrollable contractions that sent me out, then back into the stall again. When I didn't return to the table, Katie had gotten worried and searched to find out where I was. She found me sitting on the curb near the restrooms and could tell that I was both mentally and physically a wreck. She gave me a hug and asked if I was alright and within her comforting embrace I could no longer keep it together. I managed to get out a "no, not really" before tears welled up in my eyes and I began to cry. It

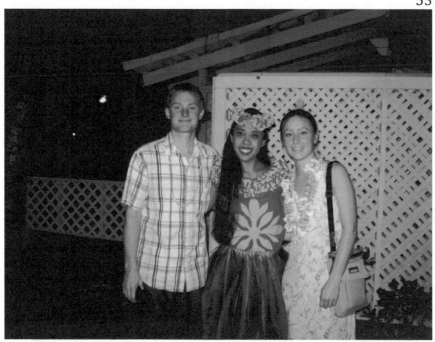

Luau in Hawaii

didn't matter that there were tons of people all around us making side-glances, wondering what was going on. I was emotionally broken and physically hurt, and I could no longer hold that in. I was tired of being something I wasn't, which was okay.

For what seemed like an eternity I remained tightly locked with Katie, trying to hold the sobbing to a minimum, but letting the tears flow. By the time I was done my face was all red and my eyes puffy. Katie's shirt was now soaked with tears but she didn't care. We created a powerful bond of understanding during those moments, in which both of us accepted each other for who we were, and how we felt, all without words.

Chapter 6

~Kauai~

We finished our time in hotel luxury on Kona and boarded the island hopper for our adventure in Kauai. The stay in Kona was one of stark contrasts. It had been a beautiful wedding, yet had been filled with anger, embarrassment, and pain for me. I was excited to move on but was equally distressed about my worsening health and the many unknowns that lay ahead. Katie and I had grown closer in many ways but in others we had begun to slip apart. The disease had become all consuming for me and left very little room for a relationship. Katie was becoming acutely aware of the intense difficulties I was setting myself up for by continuing the trip and was less and less excited about watching my intentional downward spiral. To make matters worse, the steroid prednisone was causing me to be more confrontational with Katie and I behaved sometimes like a person neither one of us recognized.

When we arrived at the small airport of the aptly named Garden Isle, the air was thick with humidity and ripe for adventure in the unknown. The owner of the farm where we would be staying, a middle aged man named Greg, picked us up and we drove up through the lush hills towards our new home.

The farm was located in a small valley that backed up to the hills on one side and opened to the ocean on the other. There was an open framed building that housed the cooking and dining area along with a small shower facility. There were four other structures on his property, one being another open framed building that had a bathroom and sleeping quarters, a yurt that was being occupied by a French couple and their baby, a wooden tent platform that housed a young lady from the states, and a teepee. The property was alive with roving chickens and ducks, two Tilapia fish farm

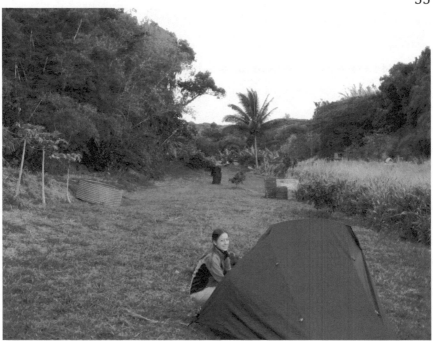

Campsite at organic farm in Kauai

tanks, avocado, banana, and mango trees, and a whole host of bugs and
insects; some interesting and some were three-inch long horror shows.

Katie and I chose to set up our small camp in a mowed area of grass
2-3 hundred yards from the main kitchen structure. Then we quickly set out
to explore the small town and capital of Kauai, named Lihu'e. The town was
filled with both tourists and locals, along with the long-term travelers like
ourselves. We spent the next few days walking from beach to beach and
around the small town. During this time, I was starting to get the feeling that
Katie was not keen on staying long term and was especially not interested in
making the valley farm our home. She was not used to the communal living
situation and was having a hard time adjusting to this new way of living. I
was also becoming aware that the farm living situation was not one that
catered very well to someone who is sick with UC. Our camp spot was a
good 2-3 minute walk from the bathrooms. It became the scene of many
early morning or middle of the night dashes. Many times I couldn't make it

that far and had to detour into the tall grasses that lay on the property boundary.

I knew from the start of the trip that the situation here in Hawaii would not be a good one, yet I was tired of always putting my disease first so I pushed my intuitions aside. I was angry that I was sick and rebellious towards the lifestyle changes that were necessary. I wanted my free wheeling life back, in which I could go here, do this, eat that, and go to the damn bathroom whenever I wanted to! I had started to put my life on hold because of the fear and unpredictability caused by the disease. I could no longer plan on that special spring break climbing trip to the desert with friends, and instead had to settle for making the decision a few days in advance based on how my body was feeling. I was tired of having UC make decisions for me and sitting back while others had adventures and grand experiences. So, when the idea of living on a tropical island came about I jumped at the idea and pushed my fears to the wayside.

After about a week of living on the farm and witnessing my declining health, Katie had had enough. She tried to suggest that we head back to the states but I would have nothing of it. We ended up staying at a nearby hotel for another four days before Katie decided to buy a ticket back home. I had to decide whether to stick it out alone or push my pride aside and let colitis win again. I decided to buy a ticket home but for two weeks later than hers. Doing this gave me confidence in my own decision-making ability and a feeling of justification for the trip itself. When Katie and I parted ways at the airport that night I had a jumble of feelings brewing inside of me. I was excited about being on my own on the misty island, yet scared to death about being alone and sick. To further complicate matters, I had given up my space at the farm and would now have to find a place to camp each night.

Katie and I left each other on good terms but with the sad feeling that our relationship may have ended. The trip, the disease, my angst, all of it had added up to a relationship that was not working. I needed time alone to figure out who I was with the addition of UC in my life, and Katie needed time to focus on her needs and wants, not just mine. I left the airport and drove north up the coast with feelings of doubt crowding my thoughts.

The immediate plan was to find a beach park on the coast to sleep for the night; somewhere that had restroom facilities and was close to Lihu'e. I had been in contact with the family friend who did construction on the island and the plan was to start work early in the morning on a house overlooking Kalapaki Bay near Lihu'e. By this point the night sky was completely dark. I drove in and around some of the nicer resorts, peered over the ocean cliffs trying to find a dark oasis, and finally settled on one of the numerous beach parks that line the coast. Katie and I had been here before and it was a nice family beach with facilities and a slightly forested area near the beach that could secretly harbor my tent for the night. Or so I thought. For those who have never visited a Hawaii beach during the nighttime hours, it can be quite the opposite experience of what it is during the day. This I would later learn is something that continues to plague the islands of Hawaii and stands as a stark contrast to what many believe to be paradise.

So there I was, short white guy rolling in a Toyota Echo with a bowel problem at midnight. I pulled into the parking area, which I noticed was a little busy for a weeknight and began gathering my camping stuff for a discreet escape into the woods. As I gathered my things, while still inside my car, I noticed that I had attracted a lot of attention from the parked vehicles nearby. Dark Hawaiian men stared at me long after I dropped my direct stare at them. I grabbed my toothbrush and headed into the bathroom to brush my teeth and get ready for bed. The first thing I noticed was the bathrooms were way too busy for 11:00pm, with people coming and going, and others just hanging out. I quickly did my thing while trying to just mind my own business, then went back out to the car. As I rounded the corner towards the car, I noticed three people hovering near it, waiting for me, or for something. I met the gaze of the three guys and said a quick "Hey," which was followed by a nod and a reply of " Are you looking for anything?" I thought about it for a second then answered, "No, I just came down to the beach to check it out and was just passing through." I quickly entered my car and decided that this was not really the best spot to grab my things and head into the woods for a good nights sleep. I then drove down a little connecting road that meandered its way closer to the water and ended at a 15-20 car parking lot right above the beach. I decided to get out and walk down the beach a bit to see if I could find a good secluded spot to spend the night. I had made it about twenty feet down the beach when I noticed a figure out of the corner of my eye, following me. I glanced back slightly while still walking and yes indeed it was someone, and, yes, they were following me. My heart started to beat faster. I clenched my car key between my middle two fingers so that it stuck out about an inch from my closed fist making a sharp version of brass knuckles. I started to circle back to where my car was parked, trying unsuccessfully to lose the strange person following me. As I continued to walk in the darkness, with the figure trailing me, I become more and more tense. I could feel the drip, drip of adrenalin jump-starting my 'fight or flight' response. In my head I am thinking "Fuck, I might really have to stab this guy in the temple with my rental car key!" I made it out of the darkness and into the light of the parking area and quickly got into the car and locked the doors. Within a minute a small, middle-aged Hawaiian man approached the car and stood nervously by my window motioning me to open the door. By this point I am both angry and freaked out so I immediately rolled down my window an inch or so and yelled, "What the hell do you want?" The man then quietly asked, "Are you looking for any action tonight?" I can't believe what I am hearing and quickly yell at him to fuck off and that I am calling the cops. He put his hands in his pockets and quickly got into one of the nearby two-wheel drive trucks and left.

I took a moment to breathe, releasing the tension that had built up inside, while at the same time trying to figure out my options for the night. I knew there was really no other area down the road, in either direction, that would offer a sleeping area, and I knew that I did not have the cash to blow on a hotel, especially the ritzy ones that were nearby. I decided to take another road that led out of the bathroom area and down the beach. As I passed back through the parking area I noticed the same three guys from before. They were off to the side of a small group of people hanging out drinking beers. They were sorting up small substances into small bags and placing them in their pockets. "Great," I thought as I drove into the darkness, a good nights sleep with prostitutes, drunks, and drug dealers. This was clearly not the perfectly safe daytime beach for kids with floaties attached to their arms and bleach white tourists in safari hats. At this point though I could not picture the tranquil scene of beach life during the day. I was preoccupied with finding a safe place to get some shut-eye before work tomorrow.

I finally found a slight pull-off on the side of the road that could accommodate 2-3 cars. I was only about 300-400 yards from the original parking area with the bathrooms but the scene was quiet, no people, and had ample camping spots tucked into a lightly treed area near the beach. The moon had come out and gave the surrounding area a nice glow. I quickly scurried into the treed area with my things so as not to be seen by anyone. Within five minutes I had set up the tent and rolled out my fleece sleeping bag. As I was sitting at the tent entrance I took a moment to look out through the trees at the beach that lay below me. I noticed a tiny glowing light in the treed shadows about 50 feet from my tent. I felt fear rise up through my body as I squinted through the shadowed darkness toward the mysterious, slightly moving golden light. I suddenly held my breath in shock as I realized that the golden light was that of a cigarette held by a medium sized male figure leaning against a tree and looking in my direction. I figured that the man was not a friendly visitor or at least not the kind of friendly I was interested in. Without moving my eyes from the man, I reached into the tent and grabbed my puny folding knife that I carry to cut cheese or fruit with. I unfolded the three-inch blade and placed it point down into the sand in front of me with one hand on it. For the next fifteen minutes I barely moved a muscle and never took my eyes off the man in the trees. He moved two or three times from one tree to the next but rarely came any closer. He repeatedly brought his cigarette up to his mouth where the golden light grew brighter then down by his thighs where it grew dimmer. It was now 1:30am. I was tired, burnt out from all of the anxiety, and sitting in the dark staring down a menace while trying to feel confident with a three-inch blade.

After about twenty minutes of the silent standoff the shadowed figure began to slink backwards through the trees. I watched until I saw him enter the lighted parking area then get into a car and drive away. I decided to stay up as long as I could or until I thought it safe enough to let my guard down. I kept watch until around 2:30am. Then, since I hadn't seen or heard anything for about 40 minutes, I decided to try and sleep. I managed to slowly drift away to the sound of lightly crashing waves nearby.

Chapter 7

~Good Days & Bad Days in Paradise~

I awoke at 6:00am and quickly broke camp. Throwing my tent and sleeping bag into the back of the Echo, I breathed a sigh of relief that I survived that crazy night. Passing through the parking area, I saw a few early morning risers, families with kids in tow, and swimmers showering off before heading to work. It was hard to look upon the beach without thinking of the very different picture of last night's events. Drug deals, sexual encounters, and possible stalking that were now replaced with sun tan lotion and sandcastles.

From the beach I drove south, back towards the town of Lihu'e, for my first day of work. As I drove, I began to worry about where I would be sleeping that night. Today's today and tonight is tonight, I thought as I pressed on down the lightly shaded road. Sunlight drifted through the leaves and vines, sending slices of light shooting into my blurry vision.

I arrived at the job site at ten till seven, met by the family friend who was nice enough to give me work while I was on the island. There were two other Hawaiians on the crew who showed me the job site and what needed to be done. The house we were working on was wedged in between two other buildings on a steep hillside, steep enough that they had hacked steps into the earth as a way to get from the bottom to the top where everyone parked. The view, however, was nothing short of amazing. The whole Kalapaki Bay stretched out in front of the house creating a million dollar vista. Surfers caught waves, tourists learned how to sail catamarans, and fishermen headed out in search of the days catch.

The work was not bad but then again it was not great. I spent lots of time doing dirt work before preparing deck footings for concrete and many hours setting up special scaffolding to which free hanging foam/concrete

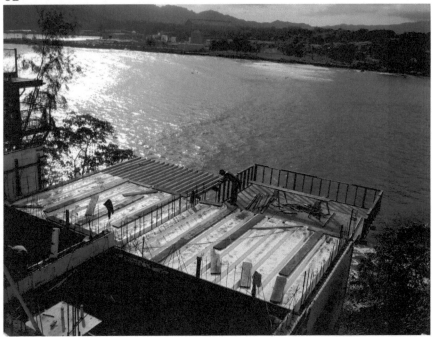

Kalapaki Bay jobsite

floors and overhangs would be built and formed upon. I was used to hard
labor jobs and had spent many hours working in construction, concrete, and
logging operations. I liked working outside with my hands but knew I would
not want to do it forever, which was why I had decided to pursue a college
education. For now though, the job was a good fit and I earned enough for
the rental car and my remaining time in Hawaii.

My UC, at this point was much calmer than when I was at the
wedding luau. My symptoms were manageable although a bit worse during
the nights and mornings but easing up throughout the day. My diet now
consisted almost entirely of cheese, avocados, and bread with peanut butter.
I broke down one day and bought a huge ice cream cone from Stone Cold
Creamery. Screw it, I thought.

I ended up working at the Bay house for three days, which earned
me enough money to last the remainder of the trip. During the three days of
work I had been staying the night at or around the job site with varying

degrees of success. The first day, when I told my two Hawaiian co-workers about my crazy night trying to camp at the beach, they all erupted in laughter and said I was lucky to be alive. They told me about the Ice (methamphetamine) problem in Hawaii and that white people in rental cars distributed many of the incoming drugs. They advised me not to camp at many of the well-known beaches nearby and suggested a handful on the northern side of the island, much too far to drive back and forth from work.

After that first day on the job, I decided I would get dinner and hang out in town until dark then return to the job site and sleep in one of the covered building spaces. For some odd reason, even though I was eating a piece of bread one or two times a day, I had resigned myself not to eat hamburger buns. One of the little hamburger joints near the bay sold a decent burger and I was able to get it without the bun, and instead get extra tomatoes and lettuce.

After my evening in town, I drove up the winding hill overlooking the bay, excited with the anticipation of a safe, quiet nights sleep. The accommodations in the building were anything but homey, yet I felt safe knowing that the chances of someone snooping around during the night were slim. I laid out my pad and fleece bag with the beautiful shadowed bay lying in front of me. Around eleven PM I began to hear the rain as it hit the foam and concrete roof above me. I fell back to sleep until I began to hear dripping in one of the corners near me. Soon there were more and more drips until the entire room turned into one big shower. In shock, I grabbed my things and ran out of the room, trying to dodge the streams of water that flowed through the various channels in the roof. How could I be so stupid to think that it wouldn't rain, or that the roof, which was mostly foam panels and far from being completed, would be watertight? I left the building, scrambled up the mud steps in the rain, mumbling under my breath how ridiculous the whole situation was. I chucked my things into the back seat of the car and jumped into the drivers seat. My hair was soaked and rainwater dripped down my face and onto my clothes. I thought to myself, was this really happening? Was I really choosing to put myself through this? With the rain continuing to pour outside I resigned myself to sleeping in the car. I put the seat back and settled into the thick, humid air and a very long night with little sleep.

My days of work were fairly uneventful and my UC condition remained stable. I was getting used to making the trek up the dirt steps to the porta-potty multiple times during the day but reveled in the privacy the little plastic bathroom afforded me. The last night, I decided that sleeping in the car was not an option again. The car was just too small and I couldn't stand the humidity. That evening I discovered a golf course directly across from the jobsite parking area, obscured from view due to densely planted shrubbery. At dusk I grabbed my camping gear and wiggled through an opening in the brush. I popped out onto a lush corner of the golf course, complete with manicured lawns and even a small fountain. Perfect. I set up the tent and within a half n hour was sound asleep. As fate would have it though, I was not meant to sleep.

At around 3:30am an explosion of hissing and gurgling woke me up suddenly. As I lay awake with my heart pounding, wondering what in the hell the sounds were, it soon all made sense. Before long the hissing and gurgling morphed into a uniformed chick, chick, chick and in a matter of seconds a forceful stream of sprinkler water hit the side of the tent. I lay there smiling, shaking my head and thinking, you've got to be kidding. Anyway, I was awake now and my colon was telling me to make a visit to my blue friend, Mr. Porta-Potty. I got out of the tent and was immediately sprayed in the face with water. Without packing anything inside or breaking down the tent I grabbed the whole thing in a giant bear hug, ripped the tent stakes from the ground and pushed my way through the brush towards the car.

Today would be my last day of work here in Hawaii and my last time fighting for a place to sleep. Tonight, I would head north towards the town of Hanalei and find a good place to set up camp, even if it meant paying for a site at one of the good beach parks my co-workers had told me about.

Chapter 8

~Resolution and a Feel for Change~

With the Echo paid up for the remainder of my time in Hawaii, which at this point was five days, I rolled into the picturesque town of Hanalei with its taro fields and quaint little shops. My plan was to spend the remainder of my time on the island exploring the numerous beaches that stretched both east and west from Hanalei and to try and hike a small portion of the famed Na'Pali coast trail. I would also try and make it to the southern town of Poipu to redeem a free surfing lesson I had received from my uncle in LA.

The beaches on the northern side of the island were beautifully idyllic; dense with lush vegetation clinging to steep mountain hillsides and surrounded with perfect blue water. I visited just about every beach along the north and east sides of the island, minus the many beaches on the north side that are only accessible via miles out on the Na'Pali coast trail. I was camping at a beach park on the western side of Hanalei for a modest $8.00 dollars a night and this suited me well.

My health condition was not getting any worse, yet it was not getting any better. I had lost a considerable amount of weight and the disease was leaving me feeling sick and tired. Most nights I was getting up five to eight times with bloody diarrhea. Sleep deprivation made me look like a zombie during the day. I was coming to the frightening conclusion that I was running out of options to manage this disease. I was on high doses of two potent medications and I was trying to follow a diet that many others swore had worked for them, yet was not really working for me. What other options did I have? Surgery? Immune suppressing drugs that cost thousands, take months to start working, and have serious side effects, such as death? The idea of surgery was becoming more and more of a possible paradise in the

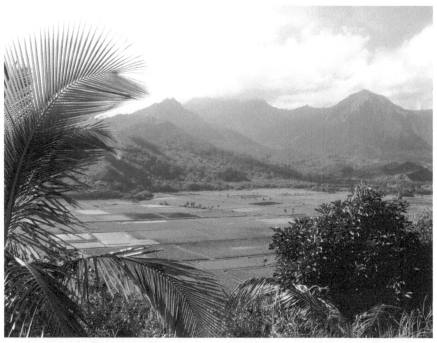

Overlooking the Hanalei valley

back of my mind. It was something that as time went on and the symptoms of UC ceased to go away, gave me comfort in knowing that I could make it stop, and stop for good. Side effects? Who cared, as long as they weren't as bad as what I was feeling now.

I was trying as best I could to eat SCD legal foods but the limited availability of food stores and cooking facilities meant a repetitive selection of ingredients, which led to binges of illegal foods. This was evident one evening when I was sick of feeling shitty, and tired of drinking warm, overpriced red wine. I went to the local gas station and did the thing I had promised myself not to do. Buy and drink beer. Dry wine is legal on the SCD but in the tropics, warm wine really loses its appeal. I came out of the gas station with a 24-ounce bottle of Corona, and proceeded to walk down to the beach and drink the whole thing. I felt guilty but damn it was good. I ended up paying for this guilty pleasure throughout the night on the toilet and resigned to never drink beer again, which to this day I have not.

My diet was still filled largely with snack foods. I rarely ate a large sit down meal, and I was not spending my money on decent food at restaurants. I was both concerned over my dwindling funds and not sure how and what to order at restaurants. I also never found a kitchen facility in which to cook a meal for myself. Both quality food and kitchen access are imperative to the diet and make travel enjoyable. It would be months before I came to grips with the changes needed to make traveling easy and efficient with SCD. For now though, I did my best but fought with the extreme cravings and gnawing hunger that never seemed to go away.

With only two days left before I flew back to Idaho, I made my way towards the northwestern end of the island where the road ends and the Na'Pali coast begins. This area is starkly picturesque and brings visions of Jurassic Park and indigenous tribes living in the bush. The plan was to hike on the famed trail for a distance, then branch off and visit Hanakapi'ai Falls, a spectacular 100-foot waterfall. The hike would be eight miles roundtrip and would test my frail body but I didn't want to miss the chance to see something I had looked at in books and magazines for years. I threw some food in a daypack, toilet paper in my pockets, and headed off for the falls.

The trail varied from dry, cracked dirt to slick and muddy. I had not been truly active in weeks and feeling my heart pumping and my body moving was invigorating. I flew up the trail as it wound and twisted along the coastline in a half run, half speed walk. The beginning of the trail was choked with tourists and hikers negotiating the trails slippery surface, both with extreme caution and excruciatingly slow progress.

I blew past most of the other hikers with a mere nod of the head or a quick hello. I was not there to make friends or to socialize but rather to view the land in its raw form and to see if I could push myself in ways I was used

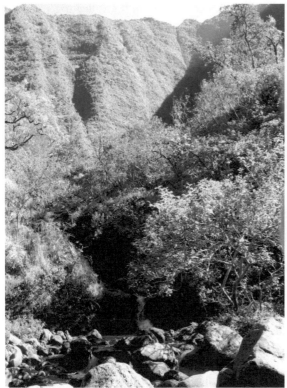
Na'Pali Coast

to doing before UC. The scenery along the trail was amazing. The rugged coastline stretched on for what looked like eternity, and the faint booming of waves as they crashed upon the beaches below filled the humid air. I was amazed at how good it felt to sweat and move my body like it was meant to do; I felt strong and in control, and it felt good.

As the trail went on there were fewer people and the environment became more rugged and wild. At the bottom of the trail where the Kalalau Trail (Na'Pali coast trail) and the Hanakapi'ai Falls trail start to head up once more, I passed a pretty little beach filled mostly with rocks. A nearby wooden sign listed a strong warning to not go swimming due to dangerous rip tides and a tally of all the people who had drowned there. Let me just tell you that the numbers were high enough to discourage any thoughts of swimming.

From the rocky 'death' beach the trail turned sharply upwards and led inland, away from the coast and into the heart of one of the many mountain valleys. The trail turned from highway style to goat path, filled with brown puddles and slick, clay mud. After about three miles the valley opened slightly and I was able to catch a glimpse of the falls up ahead. The

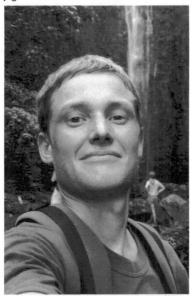

Self-portrait at Hanakapi'ai Falls

trail continued up the valley towards the towering falls, crossing the creek here and dodging into the woods there. At last I climbed up a few remaining rock and boulder sections and was presented with a view of the falls, and the dark pool it cascaded into.

There were a few other people scattered around the base of the falls and one couple swimming in it. I snapped a couple photos, ate some food, and laid around admiring the water drifting down the 100-foot rock wall. The steep rocky hillsides surrounding the falls were covered in thick ferns, glistening with the spray from the water as it plunged into the pool. I took a quick self-portrait with the camera, knowing that I would always remember this special place and headed off down the trail for the long hike out.

I was proud of myself for going on this hike and surprised at how well my body responded to the needs of my mind and heart. This experience alone would make the trip to Hawaii worthwhile. It also gave me the clarity, insight, and experience to never put my disease in front of my dreams. Not here, not ever.

My last day in Hawaii was finally here and I was all set to fly out of Lihu'e at 11pm. I had driven down to the southern town of Poipu and had made reservations to receive my free surfing lesson from my uncle's gift card. The town of Poipu was one of your typical built-up Hawaiian beach towns that catered more towards tourists and less towards the locals. Not really my favorite scene but fine to experience for a day.

I checked in at the little beachside surf shack and was measured for a long board. I was in a fairly small group of other people learning to surf, and two Hawaiian guys with safari type hats and sunglasses instructed us all. We paddled out to a small, nearby surf break and floated in a circle listening to instructions. Paddle, paddle, paddle, push, jump, and stand! After three falls while trying to get upright on the board, I finally managed to cautiously plant my two-feet firmly upon the textured board, and ride a small two to three foot wave until it eventually petered out near the shore. The feeling of riding a wave was pretty cool for sure, not something I was immediately hooked on like rock climbing, but definitely a thrilling experience.

I was still having bowel troubles like usual and even had to make a couple mad dashes from the water while surfing; throwing my board aside and running into the bathroom, desperately trying to undo the water-tightened knot holding my drawstring shorts up. I had come to the conclusion, along with the help of my mom, that when I got home tomorrow, I would make a last ditch effort to heal myself by trying the SCD 100%. Not 98% or 99% but 100% fully committed. I was excited about this prospect and being able to actually cook and prepare meals that were totally legal. I was nervous, though, that the diet, like so many of the other treatments, wouldn't work. Over the phone, I had also talked to my Grandpa Paul (my dad's father) who was out visiting in Idaho about the idea of helping him drive back east to Connecticut where he and my Grandma Peg lived. From there, I was toying with the idea of flying out to meet some friends in the climbing mecca of Red Rocks, just outside of Las Vegas, for a couple of weeks. I had not driven cross country since I was about six years old and seeing the states via car sounded kind of fun. It would also be nice to stay at my grandparent's house in Connecticut for a little while, and maybe even find a way to make it down to my mom's mother, Sue, who lived in Norfolk, Virginia. Before anything though, I wanted to make an appointment with my

G.I. doctor in Coeur d' Alene to get a status update on my condition and to make sure my body was functioning as it should with the medications I was taking.

I did my duty as a good citizen and returned the rental car on time and in good condition. In all honesty, I was kind of sad to see the little rice burner go, having had so many good and bad memories taken place in or near it. I also made sure to arrive nice and early to the airport like they say to do, even though I passed through check-in and security within fifteen minutes, thereby leaving me with an hour and forty-five minutes to stare at the wall.

The flight from Kauai to LA was uneventful for the most part, despite the fact that I, along with the rest of the passengers, thought we would plummet from the sky and sink into the Pacific Ocean.

Within minutes after takeoff we became acutely aware that the plane was flying right in the middle of a turbulent storm. The plane would shake violently up, down, and to the sides. The view out the windows looked like something out of a movie, with the clouds rushing by, illuminated by the blinking wing lights. Water smeared the outsides of the windows and the plane continued to shake. People throughout the plane began to get sick, desperately rummaging through the seat pockets for a barf bag. Others on the plane began to cry as the stewardesses left the cabin and strapped themselves into their wall seats. I, who already didn't like flying, and could get sick from the smallest bit of turbulence, lay in my seat with my eyes closed and just breathed: One breath in, one breath out, until the turbulence stopped some forty-five minutes later.

Arriving in LA, and thankful to not be floating at the bottom of the Pacific, I was glad to be back on solid ground and to be finished with the worse plane ride I had ever endured. I still had two more connections and an hour drive to make until I arrived at my final destination of Coeur d' Alene,

Idaho, so I was determined to sleep as much as I could if the plane and weather would cooperate. I finally stepped off the plane in Spokane, Washington and was slapped with the fact that, yes, indeed it was still winter here in the Northwest during late January. My mom picked me up and we drove to my house in Coeur d' Alene, which now was shrouded with a thick blanket of snow.

 Tips

Did you used to like bagels with cream cheese? Make cream cheese by dripping yogurt then adding salt to it. Spread on your favorite SCD biscuits, and let the memories flood back.

74

Tucker Returns from Hawaii

I was at the Spokane airport waiting for Tucker's plane to arrive from Hawaii. It had been a long cold January in Idaho, filled with worry over my son's deteriorating health. Before leaving for Hawaii, Tucker was having back-to-back flare ups despite taking strong prescription anti-inflammatory medications formulated specifically for UC. We never knew when the flare-ups would end and I walked a tightrope of worry about when to give in and admit him to the hospital. Dehydration, along with weight loss, were huge concerns and we monitored them closely during flare-ups. In the midst of all these flare ups Tucker somehow thought a Hawaiian vacation was what he needed.

At this time, Tucker was following the SCD with about 70 percent adherence and we both expected some relief or a lessening of symptoms to happen, showing us that the diet was working. Similar to reducing your caloric intake a little bit and watching the scale go down slowly; you see results, get motivated and reduce your calories even further. It was hard for Tucker to give up so many of his favorite foods on the SCD, plus carbs are so darn convenient to eat, so he devised his own plan combining several types of diets. The SCD takes a lot of preplanning along with a major lifestyle shift including avoidance of certain situations especially in the beginning. Going to a Chinese or Mexican restaurant while strictly following the SCD is a recipe for disaster, they are best avoided as if you are an alcoholic and avoiding the bars.

So many total lifestyle changes left Tucker sitting on the fence unable to jump off in any direction. Just when he'd had enough of this disease and was ready to commit to the SCD his symptoms would ease up and he'd feel better and lose his willpower to strictly follow the diet.

All fall and into winter, a lack of sleep and constant cramping pain with bloody diarrhea played havoc with Tucker's mental state. During these bouts of illness he found it hard to see any hope of having a life without pain or being farther than 20 feet from a bathroom. Was this as good as it gets? Was this what would define his life? Luckily, I am an optimistic person and managed to find glimpses of hope where he could see only darkness. At times though, even I found it hard to envision a normal life for my son, but I kept these thoughts to myself and continued to silently cry in the shower or during the quiet hours of the night, letting my pillow absorb the flow of tears.

I made Tucker promise to tell me if he ever felt like ending his life and talked to him about holding off on surgery to remove his colon. Tucker would research colon surgeries online, both partial ones and also full removal of the colon, and what it was like to live with a bag. I felt like this was jumping the gun and would result in a decision that couldn't be reversed if a cure was found. I strained my intuition to keep tabs on his mental state by listening closely during our phone calls for any signs of true depression or hints that he was nearing the end of his ability to cope with life, yet he remained strong and committed to life no matter what it threw at him. I learned that my fears of Tucker ending his life were my fears, not his thoughts, and I realized that my son's research into surgical removal of his colon gave him a way out of his misery and was a comfort to him knowing there was a "cure" out there if he ever got desperate enough.

Tucker had left for Hawaii at the beginning of what was to become a full-blown flare-up while surrounded by tropical beauty and the wedding of his girlfriend Katie's, sister. After the wedding, plans had gone awry between Tucker and Katie and he had been travelling alone on the islands for weeks. I had spoken to him a couple times over the phone and I knew he was struggling with some very real demons in his life. Desperately trying to find answers to the "why me" question. I still had nightmares that he would slowly waste away and there would be nothing we could do to stop the progressing disease. I laid awake at night thinking of him curled up in a tent, constant cramping and diarrhea debilitating him to the point he was unable to get out of some remote jungle campsite to find food and water. I had quieted my imagination, as I knew Tucker needed to hit rock bottom in order to reclaim his life on his terms. Don, our friend with UC, had predicted this scenario and there was nothing to do but let him ride it out by himself.

The diet takes such hard work and dedication that for some, there has to be no other alternative. You either commit, or you have surgery, uncontrollable symptoms, or possibly die. The ability to monitor or prevent Tucker from cheating on the SCD could not effectively rest with me. He had to choose to embrace the diet and follow it faithfully, not because he wanted to, but because he had to.

Ride it out he did, and now he was ready to commit to the SCD plan one hundred percent. He had called me while still in Hawaii, giving me a list of items to get and groceries to buy. We were on a roll and I was energized to begin helping. I got online and bought a yogurt maker, food dehydrator, a small ice cream maker, SCD cookbooks, and of course lots of almond flour. I added these items to my already well-stocked kitchen. I loved to cook and felt prepared to take on the SCD. I quickly reread, Breaking The Vicious Cycle, and started baking.

Now, as I stood sipping a hot cup of coffee from the airport restaurant, I wondered if Tucker would stick to the SCD plan and if it would work as miraculously for him as it had for Don. I said a silent prayer for strength and peace about the future. Come what may, I hoped my son could somehow summon the energy to keep trying no matter what.

His plane soon touched down, and tan well-rested vacationers walked past as I waited for a glimpse of my son. Tucker looked shockingly different from the other healthy tourists arriving home from the Hawaiian Islands. The disease had once again taken its toll on his body. The long flight combined with little sleep over the last few weeks had given him the look of a concentration camp victim. His thin frame, gaunt face with sunken eyes and slightly stooped posture was a look I had seen before. I gave him a big welcome home hug and silently prayed once again that the new diet would transform my son back into his healthy vibrant self.

 Tips

It's much easier to focus on what you can eat rather than what you can't!

Chapter 9

~New Beginnings~

I was able to see my GI doctor within the week and did the usual round of blood tests, all of them normal. I met with the doctor who spent a grand total of about five minutes asking about my symptoms and how the medications were working. I told him that the meds were having little effect on me, to which he replied that if I wanted, I could try just taking the Prednisone and forgo the Asacol. I told him that I had started a diet called the Specific Carbohydrate Diet to manage my symptoms and that I was hopeful of its effectiveness. His only reply was that he had never heard of it and that I shouldn't worry myself with diet restrictions and complicated food preparation because UC and diet have nothing in common.

I was confused at the lack of interest my doctor displayed about a diet that so many had sworn worked. Why would he not even look into it or tell me to at least give it a try? It was at this appointment that I decided to stop seeking approval from my doctor about my diet and to instead just rely on him for what he did best, which was to pass meds and draw my blood to make sure the pills weren't damaging my insides.

Most doctors are not trained in the art of prevention, and are instead taught how to effectively diagnose and treat disorders after the fact. I learned that seeking information about the SCD from a doctor was no longer an option because most doctors do not even know about the diet, nor have the time to research it. Trust your own instinct's and most importantly your results. If it works, stick with it.

After getting the green light that nothing unusual was going on with my condition, I made plans to help Grandpa Paul drive back east in five days. I would stay with my grandparents in Connecticut for a week then fly down to Norfolk, Virginia for three days to visit my grandmother, Sue. From there

I would catch a one-way flight to Las Vegas where I would meet up with friends Kale, Lori, Lewis, Amy, and Jeff. After spending about ten to fourteen days in or around Las Vegas rock climbing, Kale and I would then drive back to northern Idaho.

After the doctor visit I packed my things and headed up to my mom's house in Bonners Ferry, which is about a two-hour drive north from Coeur d' Alene. There I would stay until Grandpa Paul and I left for our cross-country voyage. When I arrived at my mom's house, we went straight to

 Tips

Hard-boiled eggs make great travel food for lunch, car rides or outdoor trips. High protein, quick to eat, and travel stability make them a great food!

work grabbing the SCD by the horns. Mom was alarmed at my withering condition and was ready to throw herself, and me, at the diet. She had made a batch of the 24-hour yogurt using a newly bought yogurt maker and had prepared various other treats and breads utilizing almond flour. We read through BTVC yet again, perusing the recipes and trying to understand the science behind the diet.

When I think back on this time, I remember the feelings we both had of wanting to learn and understand the scientific nature behind BTVC. It is only now, after years of science classes and experience with the diet, that I feel I have a good grasp on what is detailed in the book and why it makes sense. Don't feel that you have to understand everything all at once. If you are planning on following the diet, you really need to read the book even if you do not understand everything the first time. It would be like being a devout Christian without having ever picked up the Bible; you need the BTVC book to learn the framework and inner workings of the diet. We found most of the recipes to be easy to work with and some that have become solid weekly standards.

My mom researched beyond the book, looking on the Internet for other SCD recipe sources. I remember fondly one day, after making a trip to town for groceries, I came home to find my mom browsing through a stack of recipes she had printed off. The stack must have stood a foot tall! During those five days at Mom's, while starting

Tips

Keeping your cooler cold for long periods of time doesn't have to be hard. Place a frozen gallon jug of water into the cooler. The frozen jug last a really long time, and when it melts you can drink it!

the true diet for the first time, I tried to eat simply and wholesomely. I usually had yogurt or eggs in the morning, cheese and soup for lunch, a big dinner of meat or fish with salad, and yogurt for dessert. My hunger, due to my previous malnutrition and the side effects of Prednisone was ferocious and astonishing to anyone who was there to witness it. Three plates of food, two bowls of yogurt, and I would still be at the fridge twenty minutes later scrounging around for something to eat. It is interesting to note that the main side effects I experienced from Prednisone were: hunger, moon face, constipation, and irritability. I felt lucky about this because I had heard horror stories of Prednisone side effects like nightmares, sweating, and migraines.

At my mom's house, I started to feel as though my body was on the mend, something I had not felt for a very long time. This remission felt different. It felt like a new start for my health, instead of just a lull in my disease. The massive amounts of food I was consuming were actually sticking to my bones instead of passing straight into the toilet bowl. I had been through multiple remissions before, but this time my head felt clearer and my body stronger and more capable of true healing.

In anticipation of my upcoming trip, Mom and I set about getting prepared SCD style. We baked cookies, breads, and muffins, made our own jerky on a dehydrator, hard boiled a dozen eggs, and made a fresh batch of yogurt. This stockpile of food would last me during the trip east in the form of snacks and extras, while at dinnertime, Paul and I would choose a restaurant that could cater to my needs. For breakfast I would eat fruit, muffins, or yogurt, and I could always order scrambled eggs at a diner if need be.

After only two weeks in Idaho, Paul and I set out for our four-day crossing of the U.S. Along with us were Peg and Paul's two dogs, two newly acquired SCD cookbooks, my yogurt maker, and a cooler full of SCD goodies. We drove during the day and at night pulled off at hotels to rest. For dinners we usually chose restaurants that would carry high protein choices like burgers and steaks. My typical meal would consist of a steak, seasoned with only salt and pepper, then a salad with oil and fresh lemon juice. I was now committed to taking no chances with random, unknown ingredients like run of the mill balsamic vinegar and was happy to choose something fresh like lemon wedges. After the meal I would no longer browse longingly through the dessert menu, but instead, I thought of and waited for the lovely treats that awaited me back in the car.

Day by day we drove and ate our way across the states, dealing with good food here and bad food there. Never though did I let my commitment to the diet waver. I was stern about my needs and investigative about my food choices. This was serious, and I was serious about it.

As the slow journey from one coast to another took place, I started to have another bowel symptom that I had not yet experienced; I became constipated. I was in the middle of reducing the Prednisone down to a maintenance dose and was feeling pretty good. It felt as though the diet was not so much reducing the symptoms of UC, but rather increasing the effectiveness of the meds, so much at this point that I started to not have a BM for multiple days.

For someone who had to practically live on the toilet at times, the feeling of constipation almost felt like a stroke of luck. As time went on, however, the discomfort associated with the constipation began to feel less like a blessing and more like a punishment. It was as if the diet had given Prednisone such increased effectiveness that it had literally shut down the workings of my colon and ceased the normally overactive peristalsis that usually took place. Either way, I was gaining weight instead of losing it, and the blood in my stool had stopped. I was content.

After three nights and four days on the road we finally arrived in the quaint town of Sharon, CT. Grandma Peg was happy to see us all and was glad to have the energy of her dogs back at home. It was nice to be finally out of the car, and I had fun re-living many of the wild stories I had experienced while in Hawaii.

The next day, Peg and I went about browsing through the cookbooks I had brought and making out a grocery list for the next week. Peg did a great job of adapting to the many changes that the diet required and continued to ask many questions and offer up suggestions and substitutions.

Fully explaining what you can and cannot have while on the diet is a tough thing to do. Take sugar for example. Most people understand that you cannot have plain table sugar but then you have to add in all the other types of sweeteners like: sucralose, maltodextrin, lactose, maple sugar, brown sugar, organic sugar, etc., etc. People get confused when you tell them that you can have naturally occurring fruit sugar and honey because they are a monosaccharide (single sugar molecule) and the other illegal sugars are either a disaccharide (two sugar molecule) or a polysaccharide (multi sugar molecule). At this point their eyes have glazed over and you usually end up back at square one.

Putting the scientific version of how the diet works aside, I found it easier and less heart breaking for the person listening to list all of the things I

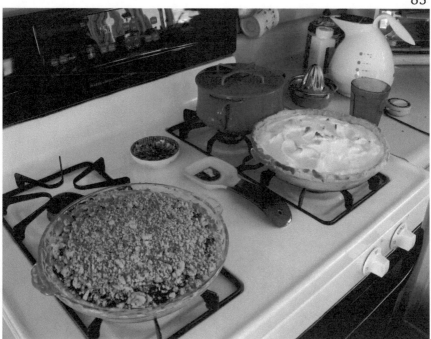

SCD pies at Peg and Paul's

could have. Foods like…homemade yogurt, baked goods with almond flour and honey, most cheeses and fruits, and a whole host of vegetables and meats. Letting people know what you *can* have, instead of what you *can't* seems to lessen the pressure and keep things simple. Especially for caring grandmas who worry you're too skinny and can't eat anything.

During the week I was in Connecticut my grandparents and I cross-country skied, visited museums, and cooked our heads off. We even got adventurous and made two pies to celebrate my birthday, a lemon meringue and blueberry crumble. Both were time consuming, yet delicious and totally worth it. I met up with one of my aunt's friends who took me to the famous climbing area of the Gunk's in neighboring New York State.

I had not been climbing in months, and it felt incredible to scale the pocketed walls high above the leafless trees below. At the top of one of the climbs, I snapped another self-portrait of myself, face full from the

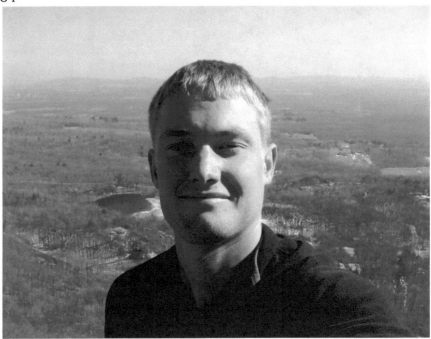

Climbing in the Gunks, NY

Prednisone, yet feeling good. Would this be a photograph I looked back upon years later and think to myself, "This is when things started to look up," or would it be a glimpse of yet another failed attempt at health? I didn't know what I thought at this point, but I was happy to be there and looked forward to the adventures that lay ahead. Nothing more, nothing less.

I finished my time in Connecticut and boarded the plane headed to Norfolk, Virginia. I had a newly stocked supply of SCD food, my trusty yogurt maker, and the rest of my belongings. I was set. Once in Norfolk I toured the city, which was where my mom grew up, and where I was born. I tried to keep up with my always-active Grandma Sue and even managed to make and eat a batch of yogurt during my three days there. The next step on my journey would entail meeting Kale and company in Vegas, then climbing until our fingers fell off, a very stimulating prospect indeed!

Besides being a great climbing partner and friend, Kale also provided a very important role in the network of friends I was enlisting to help with my new dietary lifestyle.

Kale was coming from Bonners Ferry, so I had him meet up with my mom, who loaded him up with a cooler filled with essentials. Yogurt, vegetables, eggs, jerky, and baked goods were the request, and like always, Mom came through. On this trip I would also have the luxury of being able to cook on a camp stove, drive to a grocery store when needed, and have a cooler to keep perishables fresh, something I did not have in Hawaii. I was also extremely lucky to be surrounded by great friends who, rather than judge and separate themselves from my diet, instead jumped right in and ate many of the same meals I did. And why wouldn't they? The meals we were preparing out there in the sticks were gourmet. Not some freeze dried noodle mess but instead huge stir-fry's filled with fish, beef or chicken, rounded off with a host of garden fresh vegetables.

This was the first time while away from home that I felt unrestricted while following a restricted diet. I felt I was able to accomplish this because of thorough planning, a network of friends and family, and the acceptance of the diet for what it was, not for what I wanted it to be.

It had been weeks now since saying goodbye to Katie in Hawaii, and I was longing to call her. Was she thinking of me or was she glad to get away from me and my problems? I was too unsure of her feelings and resolved to leave her number un-dialed, instead filling my time with friends and climbing.

During the days climbing, I would toss some nuts, jerky, and cheese into my daypack and this seemed to hold me over just fine. I was also able to find pure fruit bars that were SCD legal, and these provided an easy, pre-packaged method of food preparation. Hard-boiled eggs are another great camping food that is easy to prepare with a pot of water and heat, and are filled with nutrient dense protein that store well. With a hard-boiled egg, some sliced cheese, and an avocado you had yourself a meal friends would be jealous of.

Throughout the twelve days we remained in Nevada; we climbed in two different areas on two different types of rock, relaxed in slot canyon hotsprings, and renewed friendships that will last a lifetime. For me, this was a time of important personal growth, and a time to reflect on and reaffirm the new lifestyle I was getting into. The last two weeks had been game changers for me. I was feeling better than I had in six months and my optimism had gone from the dumps to my dreams. I was finally able to think about what I wanted to do and accomplish, beyond fighting this wretched disease. I was feeling the full benefits of the diet, and at this point was completely committed to it.

Kale and I reached the end of our time in Nevada and said our goodbyes to our friends as everyone headed their separate ways. We drove all through the day and into the night, soon reaching the snowy corner of northern Idaho, yet again.

 Tips

Avocados make great travel food. Pack them when they are still hard so they travel well, and then eat them when they become soft and ripe.

Connecticut Trip

Tucker and Grandpa Paul were packed up and ready to roll. Two dogs, each hanging out a window in the back seat and a huge cooler packed full with SCD food, it was time for them to head to Connecticut. I waved goodbye, leaned against the door and breathed a sigh of relief. Tucker was on his way to each of his grandma's houses and now they could cook for him! I was exhausted from cooking so much food for the trip, pretty much every pot, pan, mixing bowl, and utensil in the house was dirty. Good grief! It was a full time job just cooking for Tucker's steroid fueled food needs and I needed a break! His appetite was awesome to behold, but we all cheered for him as we saw the weight start to come back on his skeletal frame.

This diet required lots of prep time, as everything needed to be cooked from scratch. A quick jar of spaghetti sauce over pasta or tortillas with beans and cheese were things of the past. I felt like I was preparing a Thanksgiving dinner every day plus breakfast, lunch and snacks all using basic ingredients, no boxes, jars or mixes allowed!

A typical day might include a cheese omelet topped with homemade salsa and a fresh fruit smoothie swirled with homemade yogurt for breakfast. The Prednisone made him want to gorge on food again, oh, about an hour later, so second breakfast was a little more casual with a pile of homemade SCD muffins accompanied by a perfectly ripened banana. Meanwhile, a chicken with carrots, celery and onions was happily baking in the oven for lunch. Salads were made and consumed, and vegetables by the bushels were chopped for soup or side dishes. Thankfully we had a garden full of veggies and a chest freezer full of meat.

My husband Steve and I, along with my fifteen-year-old son Dylan lived ten miles from town so we kept a lot of staples on hand. As soon as lunch was devoured, I began preparing a meatloaf and snapping green beans for dinner. More homemade muffins prepared with almond flour were slipped in the oven to bake for half an hour, and I also needed to make a salad dressing again. We ran a dishwasher twice a day plus washed the big pots and bowls by hand. Everyone pitched in, but the majority of planning and cooking each meal fell to me. Tucker was gaining weight, his strength was returning, and I was trying to make this new diet look effortless so he wouldn't be overwhelmed by this different lifestyle. After all, he'd have to cook it all for himself soon enough.

Even though it felt like a monumental effort in the beginning, it was truly a joy to participate in my son's healing process. I couldn't believe how quickly he was responding to the diet. After only a couple of weeks he was feeling stronger and had a ravenous appetite. Of course he was also on a strong cocktail of steroids mixed with potent anti-inflammatory drugs, and we were glad he had them to quickly stop the destructive attack on his colon. The diet, though, gave me a sense of a long-term solution and hope for a happy, normal life for Tucker.

After he and his Grandpa were on their merry way, I got the first of many phone calls from the Grandmas. "What can he eat again?" was the usual trembling question. They had both worried from three thousand miles away as I had given many tearful reports of Tucker's declining health over the phone and then became hopeful, as I had described his miraculous recovery using the diet. Now, their precious grandson was barreling down the interstate towards them and his health was in their hands through the meals they prepared for him. The simplest way to help them understand his needs was to set them up with a meal plan for the first day or two, Tucker could take over from there. I suggested they have a gallon of whole milk (so he could immediately make yogurt), eggs, cheddar cheese, baked chicken, hamburger patties or fresh fish, green beans, salad ingredients, olive oil, a lemon and fresh fruit available for the first day or two. I tried to keep their grocery list to less than ten items so they could see the simplicity of the diet and not feel overwhelmed. It was easier to explain what he could eat, rather than go through the long list of what he couldn't eat.

I want to stress that while the diet is overwhelming to plan and implement in the beginning, it's only because everything is new and usually the person you are cooking for is still sick. Having to cook everything from scratch has something to do with it too! I constantly had to look up foods to check if they were legal for the SCD meal, I never have to do that anymore. Gourmet meals are delicious looking in the cookbook pictures but stick to simple meals at first especially if you are used to defrosting something from a box.

Tucker was also travelling with his own SCD stash of nuts, cookies, muffins and his favorite caramel nut balls to supplement in the snacking department at each house. They all had a great time visiting, and with a little preplanning, mealtimes went smoothly. Everyone ate the same things for dinner so he didn't feel like he was left out or needed to be treated with kid gloves. I think that is an important concept to understand; after all, it's a very healthy diet for anyone.

I had about a week's rest before it was time to crank out some more SCD foods for Tucker. He was flying to Las Vegas from Norfolk, Virginia to meet friends for a rock climbing adventure and needed a food resupply sent with his climbing partner Kale. Kale was driving down to Las Vegas from Bonners Ferry so we agreed to rendezvous in the library parking lot at six o'clock in the morning. I got busy making yogurt, beef jerky, pickled hard-boiled eggs, SCD muffins, cookies, crackers and lots of caramel nut balls to share. I pulled in as Kale was rearranging the back of his van to accommodate my box of food. It was a pitch black, cold morning, but I still felt a rush of warmth and gratefulness flood my senses. Tucker was feeling strong enough to participate in this rock-climbing trip with his friends. He was leading an active life again! It was hard to believe he had been so sick just a month ago.

Kale had brought a cooler full of vegetables for Tucker from his mother's market garden supply, even though it was the dead of winter. I burst into tears at the sheer generosity and understanding Kale had for my son, his best friend. He wore his gentle smile and gave me a big bear hug as he quietly said, "Everything's going to be okay, Tucker is going to be okay." I cried the whole way home thinking about all the amazing and supportive friends Tucker had rallying around him. They helped him understand that no matter what, he would always be a part of their adventures. Kale was more than a good natured, kindhearted friend; he was one in a million.

 Tips

Buy two containers for your yogurt maker. This allows you to start making one batch before you are done eating the first. Sometimes you can find a correct size jar at your grocery store in the pickle aisle, etc.

Chapter 10

~A visit from an Old Friend~

Winter turned into spring, and I was hard at work at a house North of Bonners Ferry doing some finish carpentry. I had been symptom free for two and a half months at this point and had suffered only minor instances of diarrhea or stomach pain. Nothing that resembled a flare up. I was over a month completely med-free and it felt good to no longer have the crutch of Prednisone coursing through my body. I felt as though I was right on track with the other reports of fellow SCD followers and thought that as long as I stuck to the diet 100% everything would be ok. I had made contact via e-mail with a friend of my grandma's who was also following the diet, and had been symptom free for many years. The same scenario of symptom free life after starting the SCD seemed to be the word on the Internet as well. The general word being: as long as you eat legally on the diet you should have very limited flare-ups or none at all.

Well, during that spring I did have a flare up, and it was not a little one. I remember having to visit the jobsite Porta-Potty more often and thinking, hoping, it was just some bad food or a random stomach bug. Deep down however, I knew that it wasn't just some bug, but that it was UC coming back for round two. I tried to fight it by going back to the diet basics like chicken soup, eggs, and lowering my amount of honey intake but all of this just eased the symptoms but did not shorten the duration. I tried not to become depressed about the whole situation, but it was hard not to feel down about something when you put so much effort and time into it, yet keep seeing failures.

I felt reassured by BTVC's comment that some people experience a flare up after being on the diet for two to three months, so I tried to think positively about my situation. Was what I was going through normal? It sure didn't sound like it from the conversation I'd had with fellow SCD'ers. My mom reassured me that I was on the normal course of things and that diseases like UC take time to heal.

At the time I was working as a construction framer in Bonners Ferry. I would drive up from Coeur d' Alene and stay for the week at my mom's house then return to Coeur d' Alene on the weekends. I was working with a climbing friend named Aaron during this time, and it was his dad who owned and operated the construction business we were working for. We were working on two houses simultaneously and the work was hard, yet enjoyable. Work was a steady five-day week commitment, and the upcoming holiday of Memorial Day sounded like a good break to go climbing somewhere. A couple days prior to Memorial Day, during which Aaron and I had planned to go climbing in Montana, I began to experience left side pain and a more frequent need to visit the bathroom. Then the flare-up began. My BM's went from firm to loose, to mucus, then to watery blood. I became fatigued and tired while working and almost passed out on a couple of occasions.

Once again I returned to the old ways of putting my disease in front of my plans. I called Aaron and told him that I would not be able to go with him to Montana, and that instead I would need to rest up. In reality, resting up meant curled in the fetal position all day with horrendous abdominal cramps and rushing to the bathroom twenty to thirty times, day and night. I couldn't believe I had gone from doing so well, then back to square one, all within a week's time.

My mom had not witnessed the beginning stages of a flare-up due to initial symptoms always first starting up at my home in Coeur d' Alene. She became scared and worried for my health, and nervous about the weight I was rapidly losing each day. It truly amazed me how fast the weight could come off during a flare-up. Within the first week I would quickly drop from 140lb to 125lb, and from there down to my lowest weight of 121lb. The week went on and the flare-up continued to rage within my body, showing no signs of stopping.

My younger brother, Dylan was also there to witness my declining health. He showed great patience and understanding of my condition, and for the time that our mom needed to spend

 Fact Check

Total product revenue for Colazal was $59.8 million for the first quarter of 2007.[2]

with me. Everyone at the house would always joke about the large amount of time with food preparation that mom would put in before my arrival for the week. "Wow, why don't you cook for me that way?" they would chuckle. I am sure Dylan also had to wrestle with the fear of wondering if he would be next on the UC tick list. Would he have to go through the pain of this disease, the constraints of the diet? I could only hope the illness would stop with me.

I was able to talk to my boss, Mike, and informed him of my situation. No doubt about it, I needed an additional week off. Not wanting to take more time off from work, thereby losing valuable summer money and letting my co-workers down, I decided to make the call. Within minutes of calling my GI doctor, I had secured a refill of Prednisone, and a new prescription for a drug called Colazal. I was not psyched about ingesting a new slew of medications or paying for them, but the idea of remission had me rushing to the pharmacy. I was hoping that the addition of a new medication like Colazal would provide an immediate cessation to the symptoms, much like Asacol had during its first use.

By the end of the next week I was finally able to return to work as long as the Porta-Potty was close by. I again noticed that the medications seemed to work more effectively while I was on the SCD and that my body rebounded more quickly. Symptoms of the flare-up lasted about four weeks then began to gradually lessen. The water and blood would gradually turn to mucus, the mucus would turn to loose stool, then the loose stool would become a normal stool, accompanied by three to four days of constipation.

I had been on the diet for approximately five months at this point and my commitment level was still 100%. My cravings for illegal foods were still intense but nothing compared to the yearning of prior months. Looking back I would say if you can remain 100% for three months, you should be in the clear. The cravings dropped off dramatically after the three-month mark and became more of an annoyance instead of a full-blown infatuation.

Prior to the three-month mark it was hard to even be in the same room with someone who was eating illegal foods. For me, sweets were easier to forgo, while salty and starch rich foods like chips, bread, and cereal were the hardest, especially when their aroma's filled the air. At times I would make myself crazy by holding the illegal food in my hand and smelling it; breathing in the flavors and flooding my memory with the taste.

After three-months though, these cravings started to dissipate, and I found it easier to be around many of the foods I could no longer enjoy. There were, however, dangerous situations that brought my cravings to treacherous levels and almost caused me to cheat. Many of these situations involved factors like: letting myself become overly hungry, having limited SCD foods available, being around others who were eating my favorite foods, and pressuring situations like parties.

As I became more knowledgeable about the diet and my own personal habits, I began to limit or change those situations that put me at risk. I tried to eat more frequently and always had various snack foods like nuts around. I prepared for situations like eating out or traveling by making sure I would have enough food, and pre-eating if I thought the selection might be scarce. Lastly, I changed my lifestyle to suit my new needs. My past life, filled with going to pubs for beer and pizza was no longer a reality, and wasn't something I wanted to struggle through.

The situation of being around friends, alcohol, and tantalizing food was too tempting of a venture, even after five months. So, I limited my exposure to those situations and didn't look back. This was easier said than done, but for me it flipped the situation from craving for all I couldn't have, to focusing on what I did have, and what I needed. A selfish move but one that I believe was key to my success.

The end of June rolled through and I was starting to decrease my meds, and my symptoms of the previous flare-up were about gone. I was still working with Aaron and Mike and we were now building a large house across the valley from where my mom lived. I was getting used to the system of packing a daily SCD lunch, and with the help of my mom, these lunches were the envy of the work crew. Most days I would pack a large gourmet salad with chicken or egg on top, an avocado, which I would just eat with a spoon, plus cheese slices, apple, and a SCD cookie or muffin. These meals not only filled me up, but also tasted great and offered an amazing amount of energy and quality nutrition.

To me, the criticisms I have heard from SCD skeptics about the diet being unsafe nutritionally are just plain unfounded. Sure, you could eat bacon and eggs every day and still be SCD legal but the majority of us eat a much more well-rounded diet. I, for one, eat more fruits and vegetables in a week than most of my friends do in a month, and my friends are healthy people! I consume plenty of calcium through cheeses, nuts and yogurt, fiber and carbohydrates through fruits and vegetables, and plenty of high quality protein through a variety of meats, fish, and nuts. Anyone who witnesses my diet will tell you that I eat well, and I eat nutritiously, end of story. Even if I didn't have UC, the switch to the SCD was a smart one in my mind. I feel and look much younger than my age, I rarely get colds and other common sicknesses, and I just plain feel better than when I was eating a regular diet. It is just funny to me that skeptics of the SCD say that it can be "harmful" due to the lack of carbohydrates and fiber in grains. I find this argument completely unfounded. I receive plenty of nutrient dense carbs, simple sugars and most likely triple the amount of fiber the average American consumes in my daily consumption of vegetables and fruit. At the same time, these critics are giving the OK to eat fast food, meat that doesn't even consist of edible animal parts, and ingredients that I cannot even pronounce! You be the judge.

There is also the argument that carbs are the only good form of energy. True, carbs are an excellent form of energy, but when given enough time, the body adapts and starts to produce energy very effectively from fats and proteins. I am a very active person and I have found that my energy levels while on the SCD remains very consistent and at a level that fuels my needs.

As the middle of July came around I was down to a small maintenance dose of Colazal and was completely off of the Prednisone. My bowels seemed finally back to normal and with that I was climbing, hiking, and working hard. During the later part of July however, I began to experience the routine of loose stools, mucus, and blood, all classic signs that I was spiraling into yet another flare-up. How was this possible? I had been vigilant about eating only SCD legal foods, I had slowly weaned myself off of the meds like the doctors said, and yet here I was about to descend into another relapse with UC.

My mom and I called and emailed friends who also followed the diet to manage UC, to see what their thoughts were and if they had had similar experiences. To my disappointment both acquaintances shared very different stories from mine. Both explained that once they got on the diet almost all of their symptoms had disappeared, and stayed away. They even confided that they cheated on the diet once in a while, sometimes with no consequence, and other times with just a little diarrhea or gas but no flare-up.

Why was I having such a hard time with this? Was the diet not working for me? Thoughts like this flooded my mind with doubt and confusion and caused me to question the diet's effectiveness.

The main thing that made me not give up on the diet was the fact that I had made it so far without giving in to temptation. If I were to give up now, it would be like going back to square one and having to start all over. Giving up was tempting but the improvements were real. Since being on the SCD I hadn't been as sick as I was in Hawaii or lost as much weight. These two factors alone made the dietary restrictions worthwhile. In my head, I believed that one bite or one lick of an illegal ingredient would be decreasing the diets effectiveness. I can only tell you what worked for me. The other thing that worked for me was to stick to the diet 100% rather than cheating like I had while in Hawaii.

With my flare-up symptoms returning, I also struggled with wanting to still participate in adventures that inspired me. I had already passed on the climbing trip to Montana due to UC and now a trip with Kale, Aaron, and Winter to the famed Bugaboos in Canada was in jeopardy.

 Tips

Use butternut squash in place of potatoes for most recipes. Cube it for soups, cut it into fries or mash it. Do what you want with it, the squash don't care!

Spring 2007

In the spring of 2007, Tucker was working as a carpenter in our small town. He was twenty-five years old, healthy and tanned from his travels. He was also excited about returning to college in the fall now that his health had stabilized.

Following the SCD for close to four months had produced amazing, positive changes in my son, not only physically but mentally as well. He felt in control of his life and was talking about his future with enthusiasm again. I was relaxing into an easy rhythm of cooking, cooking and more cooking.

As a family, we ate SCD meals weekdays, when Tucker stayed with us. All meals had carbs on the side for Dylan, my fifteen-year-old son, who was a long distance runner for his high school track team. Dylan was in heavy training mode, eight to twelve mile runs on the mountain trails behind our house translated into one hungry fifteen year old at the dinner table. After his run, Dylan needed serious carbohydrates and lots of them. Pasta with homemade pesto sauce; thick slabs of homemade whole wheat bread or toasted rice cakes slathered with butter, brewers yeast and cheese melted on top were his favorites. Tuckers too. Tucker would watch with envy as his younger brother plowed through plate after plate mounded with his once favorite delicacies. It couldn't be helped and Tucker learned to cope with intense cravings. To top it off, my husband Steve, a former logger, considers meat and potatoes the perfect meal.

A typical meal, which accommodated everyone, might be roast beef with mashed potatoes on the side and a big salad with lots of raw veggies on top. Winter squash baked fries rounded out the menu and we all typically enjoyed fresh fruit smoothies for dessert.

Working outside the home a few days a week meant my free time was completely filled with cooking and growing vegetables in our garden. A pleasant contentment built through March, April, and May. The easy, quiet rhythm of living in the country was finally back in our lives.

I felt the SCD was nothing short of miraculous, as long as Tucker ate only from the legal list, I believed he would never again experience a flare up.

Memorial Day proved to be memorable indeed but not in a good way. It was the start of a brutal flare up for Tucker, one that my mind refused to accept. I saw the imminent signs; increased gas, visits to the bathroom and bloating. I witnessed Tucker's increased anxiety and tried to neutralize it with "It's just a stomach ache," or "Maybe you ate overripe fruit."

By the time the diarrhea turned painful and bloody, Tucker was in a full blown, white knuckle, crawl to the bathroom on your hands and knees because you're too exhausted to walk flare up, and this time I was present for the whole show. Tucker would be close to passing out after a long painful session in the bathroom and I practically carried him back to his bed. I was scared out of my mind. This flare up was swift and heartbreaking.

Watching my son drop fifteen pounds in one week was terrifying and hurled us back to the beginning. What happened? Why wasn't the diet working? Rereading BTVC led us to believe this was a semi-typical two to three month response after being on the diet. I breathed a little easier, but still worried. Would Tucker end up in the hospital? He was skeletal thin and worn out. He had called his GI doctor, sadly returned to Prednisone plus Colazol and slowly started feeling better. I was afraid Tucker would give up on the SCD, but he surprisingly seemed more committed than ever. This return from the depths of hell was different; he healed faster while recuperating on meds and attributed it to being in better health from the SCD. I too felt the SCD was the path to wellness and I was encouraged by Tucker's positive slant on the whole flare up episode.

I took a deep breath in mid-July watching Tucker's weight and health once again climb back up to normal levels. The steroid Prednisone gave him an enormous appetite. I made SCD meals of almond flour breads, crackers, and pastries plus vegetables and salads swimming in olive oil based dressings and buttery sauces. Crisply grilled or roasted meats, mounds of creamy butternut squash, cheese platters decorated with fresh and dried fruits, yogurt smoothies swirled with fruit and honey all began to put muscle and fat on my thin and exhausted son.

I thrived helping Tucker by preparing enticing meals for him. Staying busy during daylight hours kept most of my panicky thoughts at bay; however, lying in bed late at night as my husband quietly snored beside me, was a lesson in gaining control of my terror. My tears quietly spilled onto my pillow as I tried to grapple with the horrors of my son's reality. This had been such a roller coaster year of incredible highs and lows with his health and the inevitable emotions that come with life changing events. Going from a busy schedule of work, college, travel and rock climbing to now having to stay mere feet from a toilet was a huge reality jolt for my son. Would Tucker's health ever balance out? How does UC manifest itself in other people especially young adults? How do they deal with what must be common problems?

I tried to encourage Tucker to attend an IBD support group but diarrhea is not a subject young men want to talk about in a group setting. Scared mothers-yes, twenty-five year old men- no.

We tiptoed through July; the disappointment of dropping out of a rock climbing trip with friends due to his last flare up was over. Tucker was once again feeling healthy, gaining weight, working hard, and looking forward to another summertime opportunity to hang by his fingernails on a sheer cliff with his peers. We were all amazed that Tucker still stuck to the SCD 100% even during flare ups. We wondered if there was something we were doing wrong that was contributing to these setbacks. Was some hidden sugar lurking in a piece of dried fruit that would negate the whole diet? Would a pattern of disease, then remission, haunt him the rest of his life? Could he ever be cured of UC and eat less restricted like the diet claims? These troubling questions were constant companions and accompanied me to work, to bed, in the garden, driving to town, taking a walk - everywhere.

I couldn't believe how calm my son seemed to be about all these ups and downs but if he felt in control of his future then I needed to trust he could handle what UC threw at him. Slowly, slowly letting go of trying to be in control of his disease (which I never was to begin with) was the reprieve I needed. Tucker was being extremely proactive with his health and I was proud of the resilient young man emerging from this whole ordeal.

Tucker began planning his rock climbing trip to the Bugaboos. We needed to dry some foods, as he would be backpacking not car camping with the luxury of a huge cooler filled with meats, fresh fruits and vegetables. Venison roasts pulled from the freezer were thinly cut, salted, and then dried into jerky in the dehydrator along with slices of apples. Almond flour crackers were easy to make and very portable plus the standard huckleberry muffins SCD style. Cheese chunks, handfuls of raw nuts with a few raisins mixed in, eggs cracked into a water bottle for the first days breakfast, and of course I made my caramel nut balls which had become his climbing friends favorite snack as well. Some yogurt for eating on the drive up was set aside to incubate for twenty-four hours and he was ready to go.

Another flare up the week before the trip had me secretly anxious but Tucker was determined and his friends stood by his decision to go. They would accommodate his health needs in whatever capacity he needed and again I thanked God for these amazing young men who were Tucker's friends. Kale, Winter, and Aaron continued to demonstrate unwavering devotion to their friend and climbing mate. It was a remarkable bond of friendship and one more life lesson we all learned from participating in Tuckers journey with UC.

 Tips

Learn how to pickle or ferment many foods: Eggs, beets, cabbage, onions, carrots, etc. They taste great, last longer, and are filled with healthy, good for you bacteria.

Chapter 11

~Climbing to Free My Soul~

Bugaboo: A noun, which means: something that causes fear or worry. To climbers, the Bugaboos or "bugs" as people call them, are a mountain range in the Purcell mountains of eastern British Columbia, Canada that contain soaring granite rock spires that pierce through white glaciers. Climbers from all around the world come to the bugs to test their skills on the thousand foot walls and clean crack lines that abound. Lucky for us the Bugaboos were a mere five-hour drive from Bonners Ferry so we could make a weekend trip out of it.

The trip date of August 3rd had already been set weeks before the symptoms of my most recent flare-up were becoming apparent. I didn't want to skip yet another exciting trip with friends, but the idea of climbing and hiking into a very remote area while being sick scared me. I quickly returned to Prednisone in hopes of fighting off the pending flare-up and ate simple chicken soup for the next few days. With two days left before our planned departure, I decided I would go. Screw it. If I had to turn around because I was sick, I would do that. If I had to hang my ass off the side of a cliff every few hundred feet, so be it. I would not let UC define what I could or could not do.

My mom was aware I was having another flare-up. "Are you sure you feel up to this?" she would ask. I would tell her, "Yes, I'm sure," and try to change the subject. I had my doubts, but I didn't want to fuel her worries as well. We went about packing the usual SCD suspects: jerky, muffins, hard-boiled eggs, fruit bars. The trip would be short enough that food preparation could be kept to a minimum, but it was different in that I would have to pack all of it on my back, instead of in a car. This made my selection trickier.

The day to head north finally arrived. We packed everything into the car and headed out just before 8:00 am. We planned on stopping for lunch near the town of Radium then continuing on to the trailhead. From there it would be a brutal two to three hour grind to the camp area of Applebee, which was in the heart of the Bugaboos. We made it to Radium around noon and stopped at a little pizza joint for lunch. I dined on an iceberg lettuce salad with half frozen mini shrimp on top that tasted like they had been in a can since the time of the cold war. During my "gourmet" feast I watched with envy as my friends dug into multi-topping pizzas smothered in cheese and grease. I don't need that stuff, I thought to myself as I crunched into a watery piece of lettuce and a cold shriveled shrimp.

Everyone finally finished up eating and we headed out for the last leg of the car journey, ending at the trailhead within an hour. Once there, we set about wrapping the car with chicken wire and weighting it down with rocks. This was done to prevent porcupines from eating at your cars rubber components like tires and brake lines. After barricading the car properly, we hefted our large bulky backpacks filled with gear, food, and climbing ropes and headed up into the mountains that loomed above us.

Two hours later we arrived at Applebee camp area and quickly dumped our heavy packs into a heap on the ground. I had been to the area three years earlier with a friend from work and had a great time climbing routes on Snowpatch and Crescent spire. This time, however, would be the first time in the bugs with Kale, Winter, and Aaron. I was excited to climb in this special place with such close friends.

The plan of attack was to first attempt the northeast ridge of Bugaboo Spire which dominated our view from camp. It would be the first time all of us would attempt this route. It was a classic climb complete with a superb position and clean rock. Because of the popularity of the climb, we would try and get a jump on other parties by waking up at 3:00am to be on

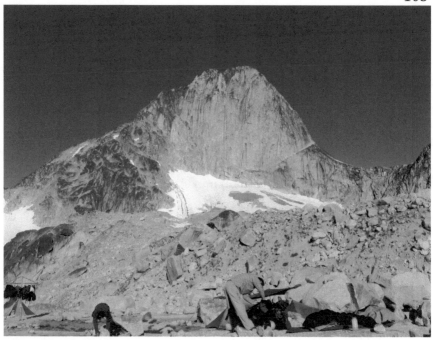

Campsite with Bugaboo Spire behind

the climb by first light. With such an early morning looming over us, we set about preparing dinner and packing our gear for the morning.

Winter had done the honor of packing a pound of buffalo burger with him, and Kale had miraculously packed a quart jar full of canned peaches. While others in the camp ate rationed, freeze-dried food packets that taste like cat food, we dined like kings eating thick, juicy burgers with peaches on the side. We went to bed with our stomachs full and our heads swimming in apprehension about tomorrows climb. My night, however, was far from being over.

The frequent trips to the outhouse began to occur minutes after finishing dinner and lasted throughout the night. I would make the long treacherous walk through and around other sleeping campers to the rock outhouse that stood on the outskirts of the camp plateau. There I would shiver and shake in the darkness as my colon passed the blood and food matter into the outhouse depths. I would then return to my sleeping bag and wait once again until I had to make the trek back.

3:00 am finally came, and I was ready to get the show on the road. I was tired of waking up all-night and sick of making the outhouse my home instead of my warm sleeping bag. I tried to choke down a muffin, but the excitement and anxiety about the long day ahead made it hard to feel hungry. We attached headlamps to our helmets, shouldered small packs with climbing gear and extra clothes, and headed off into the darkness.

The start of the climb was a scramble through a glacier filled moraine of boulders, ice and snow. Next, and still in the dark, we tackled a low angle wall that provided plenty of entertainment due to slick, un-protectable sections and falling rock, which could have resulted in serious injury or death. Once on top of the approach wall, we were presented with a beautiful sweeping, low angle ridge that gradually became vertical near the start of the climb. The top of Bugaboo Spire was just catching the first morning light, coloring the route in dark yellow warmth.

We made quick time up the ridge and soon stood at the start of the climb. There, to our surprise, were two other groups gearing up and preparing to head up the route. We unpacked our stuff and settled in, waiting for the other groups to get going before we started. The first group of two led off, then for some reason the other group in front of us said it would be fine if we went ahead of them. We quickly accepted, then Aaron and I put together our rack of gear and tied our ropes together. We decided that Aaron and I would climb as one team and Kale and Winter would follow as another team.

I laced my shoes tight and attacked the rock wall, moving inch by inch, hand hold to hand hold, in an upward fashion. I came to the end of my rope and went about setting up a belay (a belay is an anchor setup that allows a climber to attach their rope into the anchor, thereby protecting or holding a

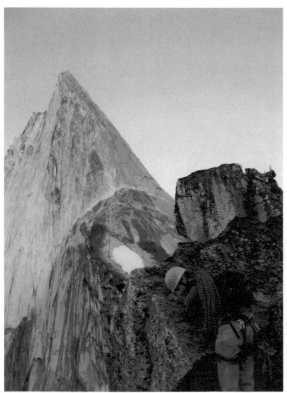

Winter climbing the NE ridge

potential falling climber). Aaron followed the pitch (a pitch is a standard length of climbing rope between 150-200 feet).

The climbers ahead of us made a blunder by going straight up instead of making a diagonal traverse up and right along a white dike. We yelled up at them that they were off route but they continued on and ended up coming back down and finishing the route in the dark. We took this open opportunity to jump into the lead and Aaron took off up the dike. We had no intentions of getting caught in the dark, high on the 10,000 foot peak, and were glad to move quickly without being held up by other climbers.

We moved up the route's many pitches, basking in the sun and marveling at the soaring spires to our left and right while listening to ancient glaciers rumbling in the distance below us. This was an amazing place and I was glad UC had not kept me from enjoying it.

My bowels had been doing fine since we started and, overall, I was feeling pretty good. I had placed a large feminine pad inside my pants in case the worst happened but in the end I never came close to needing it. The nuts, jerky, and fruit bars I had packed sustained my energy throughout the

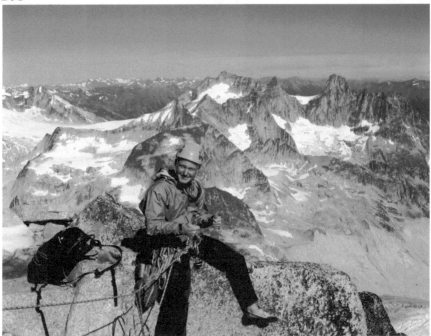

Nearing the summit of Bugaboo Spire

day, and by the time noon rolled around; we had made it to the top of the steep and technical climb. From here we had to traverse along the summit in order to reach the rappel route or way down. The traverse would end up taking more than three hours as we carefully slunk along the jagged ridge, the consequence of a misstep being a thousand foot free fall to the glacier below.

Luckily, no one fell, and we maintained safety throughout the traverse, arriving at the second summit, and the location of the descent. We rappelled down, pitch after pitch, until we were able to safely scramble across the remaining sections to the glacier below. From there, we made a quick descent of the large, steep snow chute that led down to the moraine and camp area where we had been fourteen hours earlier. Once at camp, we promptly went about eating, drinking and lounging around. We were glad to be back from the days adventure in one piece and in good spirits.

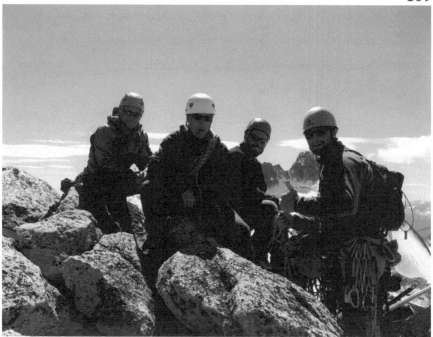

Summit! Me, Aaron, Kale, and Winter

The following day, with only one day left to climb, Winter and I set our sights on Crescent Spire with a route called Paddle Flake Direct, while Kale and Aaron decided to go climb the classic west ridge of Pigeon Spire.

Paddle Flake Direct was a four-pitch (about 600 feet) route that ascended the left flank of Crescent Spire and looked well within our abilities. I led the first pitch and soon realized that the holds I had seen from the ground were mere illusions. The gear I placed for protection was small and scarce and the climbing hard. Up a right slanting corner then though an overhanging bulge I went, all the while not sure of what to expect next. I ran out of rope right in the middle of a steep finger crack section and was forced to set up a makeshift belay with what gear I had left. I belayed Winter to my impromptu hanging belay and bid him good luck on the heinous looking wide crack that loomed above us. Winter made a few difficult steep moves off the belay and then stood face to face with an ugly six-inch crack. We had brought no gear that would fit a crack that size, and we both realized it the moment we spotted it. He looked at it this way and looked at it that way, but the crack wasn't planning on changing for him. So, Winter did what he does best, and shoved his arms into the crack shoulder deep, and commenced to climb the thing with impeccable style.

The remaining two pitches were long, easy, and enjoyable. We made it to the top, snapped a few summit poses then made our way to the rappel route to get down. By the time two-o'clock rolled around, we were back at camp where Kale and Aaron had just arrived. Both climbs turned out to be spectacular and we all enjoyed re-living the play-by-play, pitch-by-pitch, narrative of the day's climbs.

After getting a bite to eat at camp, we quickly packed up our things and started the steep, knee jarring descent back to the car. I was inspired by my accomplishments during this trip and my ability to push my fears aside and follow my dreams and aspirations. Who cares if I had to live half the night in a damn outhouse, I had climbed a thousand foot vertical wall in one day and I was proud of that. I may have headed home that day in the middle of yet another depressing and painful flare-up but I was making progress, and I realized the SCD diet was to thank for it. Two steps forward, one step back.

 Tips

Be aware of concentrated carbohydrate foods that have lots of honey, peanut butter or dried fruits. They may be contributing to flare up activity so eat them with caution and always in small amounts.

Chapter 12

~*Feelings of Doubt with a Side of Happiness*~

Months passed and the cycle remained the same. Flare-up, slow recovery, a few weeks of good health, then a slow relapse back into a flare-up. Repeat. I was growing tired of this ugly cycle, yet remained fully committed to the diet even though at times it would have been easy to lose faith. I tried my best to research other cases of people who were on the SCD and who had experienced setbacks, but could find only minor incidences.

I called Lucy, the owner of Lucy's Kitchen shop in Bellingham who is a long-term follower of the diet and was an acquaintance of the late Elaine Gottschall, author of BTVC. Lucy explained that every person has a different reaction to the diet and diverse degrees of disease progression. She said to count myself as lucky since I had never been hospitalized or hooked up to IV's for nutrition. She told me that some people bleed for years while following the diet, and it just takes time to heal serious diseases like UC or Crohn's.

Concerning the diet, she told me to be acutely aware of certain legal ingredients that may give me trouble. Some of the things she mentioned were peanut butter, too much honey, and especially the wickedly delicious peanut butter caramels that I now believe caused, or contributed to, my multiple flare-ups. Overall, she told me to be cautious with foods that gave me gas or were followed by any kind of stomach problems. The final advice she gave me was to just give the diet time and that UC takes a long time to heal.

I got off the phone with a renewed confidence that what I was doing was a step in the right direction. I was seeing positive changes, it was just that they were slow and not what I was expecting. I kept telling myself to give it time, and to count myself lucky I had never been in a hospital attached to an IV line. Two steps forward, one step back.

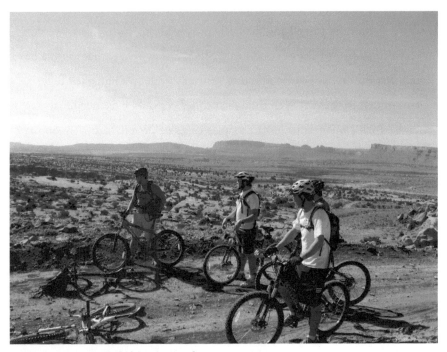

NIC group mountain biking in Moab

Throughout the winter I continued to have good times and bad times. Flare-ups came and went, but each with less intensity than the one before. By March I had managed to get through a flare-up without the aid of Prednisone and now relied solely on Colazal to manage flare-ups. Making it through a flare up without Prednisone was somewhat of a breakthrough for me because I felt it was keeping me in a cycle of relapses. At this point, I also felt that I just didn't need it anymore, as the flare-ups were more like a bad case of diarrhea instead of a crawling on the floor, knockout disease like UC. The longer I stayed on the diet, the stronger I became and the weaker UC felt.

I was now back in college at NIC, and as spring break was fast approaching I made plans with the NIC Outdoor Program to go on a mountain bike trip to Moab, Utah over the break. I worked out a deal to do all of the cooking for the group and to lead some of the rides in exchange for a free trip. I was on a maintenance dose of Colazal and was planning to reduce it to the point of stopping while on the trip. I was feeling strong and excited about heading towards the warm desert sun. I told Kale about my plans and he quickly came up with the idea of driving down to Moab to meet me once I was done with the NIC group. From there we would head farther south and go climbing for the remaining break, plus tack on a few extra "personal days".

Spring break finally came and we filled the school van full of college students and a trailer with their bikes. We left around 11:00 pm that night and drove until the following day, arriving tired in Moab around 1:00 pm. We had reserved a large house at one of the local hostels in town, and, once there quickly went about setting up the place to accommodate the large influx of college students.

I had a private room with the other instructor, which had its own bathroom and two large beds. My bowels were doing pretty well during the day and only had minor issues of urgency during the mornings. It was enough to stress me out, though, during the early morning times when bathroom space was at a premium and I was on a tight time schedule.

During those five days in Moab, we rode till our legs about fell off and our arms were burnt from the desert sun. We rode miles of slickrock terrain, in which our tires never touched dirt for the duration of the ride. Many of the rides would take us all day, and it was wonderful to be immersed in the red rock country for hours at a time. We rode many of the classic rides of the area like Slickrock and Porcupine Ridge. We also found more secluded rides into desolate backcountry filled with red rock towers and mesa views.

On the third day there, I stopped taking Colazal as I had planned and continued to ride without the meds coursing through my body. Each day my legs and body grew stronger and my mountain bike skills improved. I felt alive and youthful in the desert sun, and it felt good to be healthy once again. It had now been a year and three months since I first started the diet. I was starting to feel that my commitment to the SCD was finally paying off. Months had passed since I had experienced a serious flare-up and I could feel the disease weakening. It was not so much that I felt the SCD diet was curing me, rather it was taking the fuel away from the disease, rendering it weak.

The school trip ended, and I waved goodbye to everyone, sad to see them go, but relieved to no longer be in charge of everyone and responsible for feeding them all. Kale picked me up and we drove two hours south to the rock-climbing destination of Indian Creek. We spent two days sinking our hands into the plentiful, parallel cracks that abounded there and after that, traveled to Castle Valley with the intention of climbing on the famous Castleton Tower and Rectory.

The next morning, we hiked up towards the towers to climb a route called Fine Jade on the Rectory. When we arrived, we were greeted by four other groups waiting in line at 7:00am. There was no way we were going to wait in line, so we set our sights on the neighboring tower of Castleton. Both of us had climbed Castleton before but not via the imposing North Face. We hiked over to the bottom of the route to get a better look at the route's features. The face looked tall, hard, and scary. We both hemmed and hawed about it for over an hour. Finally we figured, why not? We were here, no one else was on it, and it was supposed to be a good route.

I racked up my gear and led up the first pitch, which was a stellar hand and fist crack that went for 200 feet and took everything I had to complete. Kale led the second pitch, attacking a wave like feature that followed a perfect hand crack through an overhang.

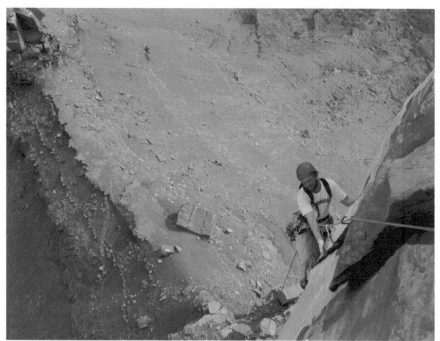

Kale climbing the North Face of Castleton

And then there was the last pitch. Both of us were at a hanging belay, our feet on a 1x2 foot ledge with our butts hanging out over space. We were looking over at the large, off-width flake that comprised the final pitch to the top, and were trying to guess at its difficulty. The slightly overhanging flake of sandstone looked manageable but the position and commitment required was truly intimidating. I knew it was my turn to take the sharp-end, and with this I grabbed the gear from Kale and started the slow traverse towards the flake above. The width of the flake was too big to jam or wedge myself into, forcing me to remain on the outside of it, lay-backing up the edge while my feet smeared on the gritty rock. Move up a couple feet, wedge a leg and foot behind the flake, pull out my biggest cam (camming units are used as removable pieces of protection while ascending routes) and shove it into the crack, take a deep breath, repeat. The ass-pucker section soon gave way to easier climbing up higher and as I came closer to the top my fear gave way to pure bliss. The last thirty feet to the top brought me back to reality as the solid sandstone gave way to unconsolidated sand minus the rock. This is the kind of stuff that you crush with your hands and looks more like mud than rock. I rigged a spider web of protection in the crumbling rock and made the final push for the sunlit summit. Out of the darkness and into the light I went, glad to be through with the anxiety filled climb and energized by the adrenaline coursing through my veins. I belayed Kale up to the summit, who along the way, just kept saying, "Wow, cool, wow!" as he climbed.

After taking a few photos and signing the summit register we rappelled back down to our backpacks and headed off to the van. Kale had brought a cooler full of fresh vegetables from his mom who operates a market garden in Bonners Ferry. We went to the grocery store in Moab and picked up a nice piece of salmon, then drove out to our desert campsite and promptly sautéed it and ate it on top of the fresh greens. This meal was so good that both Kale and I remember it to this day, and have tried on many occasions to re-create it with limited success.

The following day we drove north, heading back towards Idaho. We managed to bag another desert tower called Turkey Tower on our way north and both felt lucky to be alive after the four-pitch, horror fest the tower delivered us. We drove through the night and arrived back at my house in Coeur d' Alene in the wee hours of the morning, where Kale dropped me off, before continuing on toward Bonners Ferry where he was staying. Life resumed its normal course of events filled with school, work, and a rekindled relationship with Katie. Another thing was also different. Months had passed and UC had not raised its ugly head, I was also med free. Would it last?

September 2007. Tucker had been on the SCD for eight months now and was still having flare-ups almost back to back. He would catch his breath during a short period of perfect health; quickly gain back lost weight due to raging hunger and Prednisone, and then slowly wean himself off the medication. He would then lie in wait for the next flare up to come, as the lower realms of his body once again began the process of purging itself of all nutrients.

Tucker had returned to college in late August and was living at his house in Coeur d'Alene, so we didn't see as much of him as we had over the summer. After much coaxing over the phone about how school was going during another flare up, he admitted to not eating breakfast or lunch to deal with multiple bathroom trips during classes and tests. If he didn't eat, then he didn't have to use the bathroom. Knowing he has zero body fat on his best days, my worry barometer started rising while at the same time I knew it was the only way for him to deal with his immediate problem.

Despite his current weight loss, I was even more worried about his mental state; it seemed as if his flare-ups were finally getting the best of him. He sounded exhausted and depressed on the phone. I easily convinced him to head North to "Moms" for much needed rest, saying I would cook for him the whole weekend.

He arrived, looking very thin but not as sick as he had during previous bouts of illness. After lunch, we lounged under the long-needled branches of an old Ponderosa pine in our backyard, silently enjoying the warm fall day. I peeked at Tucker; eyes closed, relaxed, slowly breathing in the pine scented mountain air. His face was rounded, artificially full from the latest doses of steroids. With no contours of muscle to cling to, his clothes hung limply off bony shoulders. My thoughts lazily drifted to remembrances of a healthy boy living an idyllic childhood.

Tucker grew up right here, ten miles from the small, friendly town of Bonners Ferry. His early childhood was spent riding Babe, his mountain pony, all day in the foothills of the mountains behind our home. When he was twelve, he bought, with his own money, a two-year-old Arabian gelding named Sam; they bonded so completely that Sam never had to be penned behind a fence. He freely roamed our property waiting for Tucker to emerge from the house for another grand adventure on the trails that led from our backyard. It was pure wilderness surrounding us and Tucker thrived in the freedom he had to explore it. Inflammatory Bowel Disease and Ulcerative Colitis would not appear in our vocabulary for ten more innocent years.

I was jolted back to the present by the sound of Tucker trying to hold back the emotional consequences of his situation. The dam holding back his emotions since being diagnosed had sprung a leak and it was about to burst wide open. I had been anticipating this for a long time and quickly pulled my thoughts from the past to be fully present for my son and his grief. The anguish that spilled out identified the sadness I had observed earlier. Thoughts of being single the rest of his life had been haunting him. "Who would want to buy into this!" he cried out; angry now at what life had dealt him. He continued, on a roll now. "What do I have to offer someone? I'm skinny and weak, chained to the toilet, can't go out and drink a beer, and eat a weird diet."

I let him rant for a few minutes about the unfairness of it all, and then I quietly spoke. I told him it wouldn't be a silly, immature, partying type of girl he would date. They would quickly weed themselves out. Instead, he would find someone who saw him as an amazing guy, with lots of wonderful qualities, who happened to struggle now and then with symptoms of a chronic disease.

She would be a strong, intelligent, compassionate person herself, knowing that we all struggle to live the best life we can with what we are given. Living a healthy lifestyle and creating a rich home life would be important to her too. I watched as Tucker quietly processed all this. He seemed to accept what I saw in his future as a possibility for him to open up to and receive. This was another turning point in a very tumultuous year. Little did we know, that in the spring, along with the daffodils and tulips, Katie would come back into Tucker's life. She was exactly the picture of the beautiful, strong, intelligent, and compassionate person I had drawn for Tucker five months earlier.

That fall and winter were rough. Dealing with multiple flare-ups shook my son's confidence in the diet for the first time since he'd started. Having to take Prednisone every 6 weeks or so was scary on many levels for us all, and it was beginning to feel like it was contributing to a pattern that the diet wasn't able to fix. Feeling desperate, I called Lucy's Kitchen Shop and spoke with Lucy herself about Tucker's fears that the diet wasn't working. Could he be in the small percentage that BTVC talked about who did not get better on the diet? Over the phone lines I felt Lucy's confidence in the SCD (and yes, I was crying on my end) but only if it was followed one hundred percent. Once she believed Tucker was not eating any illegal foods we continued our quest to find culprits within the parameters of the legal list of foods. She first asked if he ever ate peanut butter caramels (made with a widely circulating SCD recipe) as they gave lots of trouble to many people. I knew right away we'd found the perpetrator. There was a huge pan of them in the freezer at that very moment as they were a favorite treat of his. Being aware of concentrated carbohydrates like that gave us a new vision of the SCD and as Tucker continued to ask Lucy questions I got rid of the offending treats.

Spring burst past a dark winter, the peanut butter caramels were a distant memory, and with that Tucker's health had improved dramatically. He had miraculously completed another year of college despite continuous flare-ups throughout the fall and winter. The SCD was again starving the bad bacteria as Tucker nonstop fed his digestive system probiotics in the form of yogurt and supplements.

I rarely cooked for my son anymore; he was doing just fine in his own kitchen. Luckily, he had always enjoyed playing the chef when he was younger especially creating artistic salads using colorful vegetables from our gardens. Experimenting with cooking during his childhood years was definitely coming in handy now. During Spring break he had participated in a college bike trip exploring Moab, Utah. Not only had he kept up with his own daily dietary needs while in school but he had preplanned, cooked and baked SCD necessities for the ten day venture and also was in charge of cooking for everyone else on the trip. I realized my son was going to be able to pull off this diet on his own and I've never been prouder of him. He had persevered despite confidence shattering relapses, and discovered within himself a strength that he could triumph over whatever life had in store for him. In our family, we are all better people because of witnessing this victory; it is a gift he continues to give us.

While we were astonished with Tucker's willpower, watching him follow the SCD one hundred percent, we knew it wasn't easy making so many adjustments to his diet and lifestyle, yet he did it with very little complaint. Before UC, Tucker had been quite the brewer of amazing beers producing delicious dark, creamy ales and experimenting with espresso beans, chocolate and various hops for subtle flavors.

Beer on the SCD is only a pleasant memory so he embraced red wine with the passion of a true connoisseur. It was important for him to find substitutions of acceptable foods or drinks to replace the enjoyment of previous indulgences.

The spring and early summer of 2008 were the healthiest Tucker had experienced for a couple years and we looked forward to a quiet summer. Life was slowing down to a very pleasant rhythm and everyone was grateful for the vacation from worry. My husband Steve, my younger son Dylan, and I picked up where we'd left off with our lives. Life felt peaceful again as we watched Dylan run for his school track team, and later cheered him on as he participated in his first triathlon. Tucker and Katie grew closer and planned a trip together to Mexico. Life was good and I was grateful to all the people who had helped us through the rough patches.

The SCD was working as it had been all along. We just expected instant results, like when he was prescribed steroids or other medications, but true healing takes time. Medications all have side effects, some of which present health threats themselves, whereas the SCD is a nourishing diet for anyone to follow so it's always a better alternative to medications. The book BTVC even says it takes a couple years at a minimum to heal UC symptoms but it was hard for us to envision just how those years would manifest themselves. Personally, I naively thought the moment Tucker started the SCD he would never have a flare up again. That belief clouded my vision to the point that I was unable to see the slow but steady healing that was taking place all along. Two steps forward, one step back.

Chapter 13

~Confidence Rising~

Months passed and still no flare-ups. I kept holding my breath, waiting for the usual symptoms of UC to start sneaking into my bathroom business, but they didn't. May, June, July of 2008, and still no UC. I had small periods of loose stools but they never progressed, and usually didn't last more than a week. I was still committed 100% to the diet and was pleased to say that I had never cheated (at least to my knowledge) since starting the diet in February 2007.

My diet no longer was something I dealt with, or had to work around, but instead was firmly rooted in who I was and the lifestyle I led. Incorporated into this new lifestyle was my former girlfriend Katie. During the previous month I decided to visit her at her workplace and the relationship slowly grew from there. Same people, yet with newfound perspectives on each other. I was finally able to share with someone more about myself than the overwhelming feelings of fear and disease. I was able to think and express my situation more clearly now and let go of the angst that haunted my psyche and forced me to do irrational things. My mind felt clearer and my body less damaged and scarred. I was ready to love again, and I noticed that Katie could see this. Dealing with a disease like UC at such an early stage in the relationship is hard. It puts not only stress on the individual suffering, but also on your loved ones or caregivers.

Tips

Double it, triple it, quadruple it! Increasing the portion of food you make not only saves cooking time, it also saves you the headache of finding something to eat when you've had a long day.

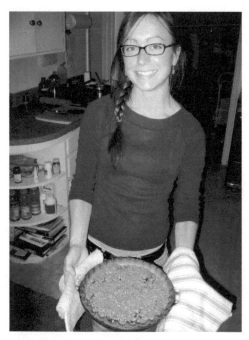

Katie the master pie maker!

Together, Katie and I embraced the way of life that the SCD diet imposes on loved ones, and together we grew stronger. With the guidance of my mom and the help of Katie, I became better at preparing and cooking the foods that nourished me. I had a continual rotation of yogurt going on the counter, soup from scratch in a matter of minutes, and a delicious meal ready to roll within minutes of coming home from work or class. I had my network of support ready in times of need and I had become used to packing for longer trips out of a backpack or car. I climbed in the Sierras of California, ice climbed in the far reaches of Canada, backcountry skied through untracked snow, and mountain biked the backwoods of Idaho. Life was good. The routine of preparing, eating, and living by way of the SCD was no longer abnormal. At this point it would have seemed weird to return to a normal diet of grains and nasty processed filler foods. I liked my diet and way of life, and I was sticking to it!

Summer turned into fall, fall into winter and time moved on without thoughts of UC. My cousin Andrew and I sold our house, as he had just found out he would now be a father, and neither of us wanted to pay the other off for the house. I ended up taking my share of the profits and buying a house nearby and spending the winter remodeling it and making it into a rental. The house ended up turning out better than I could have expected but I hope I never have to live in a house while remodeling it at the same time. It's rough.

That next July I found renters for the newly remodeled house and made plans to spend nine days in the Yucatan with Katie, followed by some time up at my mom's house. In August, Katie and I, along with our new Boston terrier named Pepper, would move south to Boise, Idaho. I would continue school there to

Tips

While preparing to travel to another country, look online for food translations and print them off. There are great resources for gluten free people, many of which list/interpret illegal SCD foods.

become a physical education/health teacher and Katie would start her career as a nurse. Things looked good and we were excited for the upcoming change.

Traveling to the Yucatan would be a big trip for Katie and I and a big test for my diet abroad. This time there would be hotels with cooking areas and money available to eat out most dinners and breakfasts. I was also more confident and wise about my diet and didn't have the cravings that would send me teetering towards illegal foods. The time frame of nine days also seemed like a good decision. Just enough time to get in, see the sights, and get out before I might get into trouble with UC.

As the plane touched down we scampered away from the dregs of Cancun and out to our island destination. We swam in the clear Caribbean waters and relaxed in hammocks strung between palm trees. Life was good. Following the SCD diet took some practice but soon became easy. We usually had breakfast at a beachside joint that served great eggs with veggies on the side. Lunch consisted of mangos, bananas, papaya, and pineapple

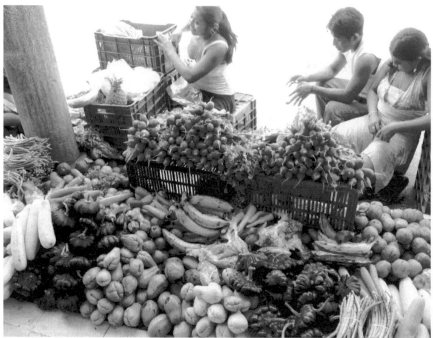

Fresh food market. Yucatan

with cheese on the side, all bought at the local market for dirt-cheap. I had also brought with me some almond flour cookies, fruit bars, and some jerky. After miraculously getting through Mexican customs I realized I had risked a fine or jail time for bringing such items into the country, especially the meat. You have been warned! Dinners out I found to be easier than most places in the U.S., due to the simple ingredients used and the lack of filler additives. In most cases I was able to dine on fresh fish, vegetable dishes with extra guacamole, minus the rice, and wash it all down with fine Tequila (I am not sure Tequila is SCD legal but in small amounts it caused me no issues).

During the second half of the trip we traveled inland toward the pyramids of the Maya and the quaint town of Valladolid. Here we took multiple trips to the ancient towns and cities of the Maya and explored the underground sinkholes known as cenotes. Here again, I was rewarded with a rich selection of SCD foods and dishes to choose from. Less seafood, and more dishes with various meats like roasted chicken and steak, along with an always-plentiful selection of fruit and fruit juices; all fresh squeezed before your eyes.

The Mexico trip opened my eyes to the possibilities of travel away from home and camping coolers, and filled me with a sense of relief that it was possible to travel this way. We finished our trip and flew back to Idaho to pick up Pepper and the rest of our belongings. From there we made our way south to Boise and into a new life.

We bought a house in Boise and Katie began work at a nearby hospital while I started school at Boise State University. My stepsister Stephanie and her husband Jon owned an oxygen manufacturing & delivery business where I worked three days a week. It was a perfect combination of enough money and plenty of time off for school. We planted a garden in the backyard and began eating wonderful meals all picked mere feet from our door. We also began visiting our local farmers market on Saturday mornings and learned about the vegetables and meats we were eating and where they came from. Food became more interesting and part of an adventure instead of just the means to an end.

Life in Boise was new, fun, and exciting. We went climbing at the local Black Cliffs area, and on weekends traveled to the famed City of Rocks; a three-hour drive east. We also explored the restaurant scene in town and found places that could easily cater to my diet and those that could not.

But as our cooking skills increased, and our ingredients grew in quality, we found that many of the restaurants just couldn't compete. Another problem with going to a restaurant was that there was very little I could actually eat off a menu. Hamburgers, salads, and steak, that about covers it. Now, you could make a laundry list of requests to the kitchen and wait-staff about your dietary needs, but in all reality, mistakes will happen and the food you end up with most likely will have illegal ingredients in it. For me, the risk in these situations is too great to endanger my health. Therefore, I stick to easy, simple dishes while ordering out: burgers minus the bun, salads with oil and lemon (unless I feel the wait-staff really knows their stuff or they go ask the kitchen about added starch and sugar). In certain situations I have even brought along an SCD bun for my burger and my favorite homemade salad dressing to top my salad. Katie is usually the instigator on these "imported ingredients" and hides the buns or salad dressing in her purse until I need it. Small things can make you feel a bit more normal, and less like a Type-A food freak.

A year after moving to Boise, I asked Katie to marry me and we made plans to have the wedding at my mom's house and property in Bonners Ferry. We set the date for July 18th and started making all of the arrangements. The big day finally arrived and the wedding site looked amazing. We had rented multiple tents, filling them with tables, and vases bursting with wildflowers that Kale's mom had grown. My dad volunteered to handle all the cooking details and made the best barbecued chicken and pesto salmon. The wedding was made SCD friendly by saving out a few pieces of chicken without BBQ sauce, and my mom whipped up a small cake with almond flour just for me. Katie and the guests had their cake and I had mine; everyone was happy. With all of our closest friends and family we celebrated late into the night, Katie and I were now a married couple. All that was left now was the honeymoon.

Katie and I had searched high and low for a honeymoon location and finally chose the British Virgin Islands (BVI's). We planned on vacationing for fourteen days and on two islands, Tortola and Virgin Gorda. This would be the longest trip out of the country I had taken while following the SCD, yet I was confident after the Yucatan trip that I would be able to find ample food options while there.

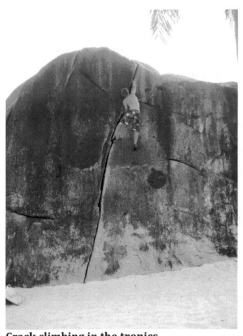

Crack climbing in the tropics

In Virgin Gorda, we stayed in a wonderful apartment style hotel. Lush palms and tropical undergrowth surrounded us and it was a short walk to the ocean. The apartment had multiple rooms and a full sized kitchen, making SCD cooking easy. The BVI's are best known as a boating destination, and boaters come ashore to buy supplies or eat and drink during the evenings. This made the island tranquil and un-crowded.

We swam and snorkeled at the famed Baths and hiked to the highest point on the island through a dense forest trail. I even brought my climbing shoes and chalk bag and climbed on the many boulders that lay tumbled about on the beaches near the Baths and Spring Bay. The rock was fabulous and contained many stellar cracks and climbing features. The hardest part about climbing in the BVI's was not the availability of rock but rather finding the motivation to do anything active in ninety-degree weather with 100% humidity.

Before coming to the islands we had researched the food scene and had heard that it was expensive, yet extremely good. The expensive part turned out to be true but the good part needed some imagination. Everyone spoke English but I found the food contained lots of additives and spices that also contained sugar. The process of trying to explain that I had serious food allergies to certain ingredients also seemed to be a topic that was lost on many a server and cook. We started to figure out that the scenery and water were amazing but the food left much to be desired.

After eight days on Virgin Gorda we boarded another ferry and headed to the island of Tortola. We would stay on Tortola for the remaining six days then catch our return flight off the island. We rented a car, and headed off for adventure part II. Tortola was much bigger than its sister island of Virgin Gorda and had the largest population of residents and tourists. We drove through the islands capital city. It was completely packed with cars and people and we miraculously made it through to the other side without hitting someone or getting into a car crash.

The hotel room we had reserved months earlier was on the opposite side of the island and sat mere feet from the calm waters of Cane Garden Bay. The hotel was fairly cheap, and it showed. Compared to our digs on the other island, and for about the same price, our new hotel was kind of a dump. It did however, have a closet kitchen complete with a small stove and oven, and a mini fridge. This was nice because I was able to buy some eggs and sugar free sausage from the general store down the street and cook up breakfast and snacks on my own.

Everyday we would pack the rental car with the days supply of food, snorkel gear, and sunscreen and take off to find and explore a new beach. Once at the beach we would go about living the hard life, which was lazing around and snorkeling until our backs started to burn from the intense sun.

Breakfast was usually eggs and a sausage patty all made in the hotel room. Lunch was snacks like fresh fruit, fruit bars brought from home, and hard-boiled eggs. For dinner we always went out to one of the local restaurants, and in the beginning this was fun. After a while though, dinners out started to become something I did not look forward to. I found that the menus at all of the places were about the same and that I was eating a modification of the same meal day in day out. The case would have been the same back home in the U.S. but here I could not have a break and eat a home cooked meal, something I desperately wanted and needed to do.

The trip was turning out to be just too long. The island was absolutely gorgeous but we had seen everything we had come to see, and even Katie was getting tired of eating the same meals day after day. The other issue was the fact that I knew I was eating illegal ingredients here and there in my nightly meals out. The rub mix here, the sauce that was taken off but still thinly remained on my food there. All of it was still incorporated into my meals no matter how hard I tried to explain my situation to the restaurant staff, and I was starting to feel the effects of it. My BM's began to happen more than once a day and their urgency began to catch me off guard. We only had two more days left so I resolved to eat as simply as I could while at restaurants and to cut down on the fruit a bit until we got home.

Our last day arrived and we dropped the rental car off early in the morning and walked over to the small airport to catch our plane home. Eighteen hours later we arrived in Spokane, WA where my mom met us and drove us up to Bonners Ferry. With commitments back in Boise we quickly packed our gifts from the wedding, threw the dog in the car, and left for the ten-hour drive home.

The symptoms of UC slowly kept progressing even after being at home and eating fully SCD legal meals. The feelings that I had recently managed to forget, returned to stir up bad memories, and this scared me. I had been symptom free for over a year now and thought I was home free. This time was different though. I knew that the culprit was the amount of illegal foods I had consumed during the trip, and to me this was reassuring. My body was simply responding to the non-SCD foods I had ingested.

The flare-up progressed to the point of bleeding but never crossed the line of being agonizing like so many in the past had been. I made it through the flare-up without medications of any kind and promptly regained my previous levels of good health. Two steps forward, one step back.

<u>July 17, 2009</u>

It was the day before Tucker and Katie's wedding and everyone bustled around our yard taking care of last minute preparations. Steve and I had worked hard all spring and summer clearing out the inevitable piles of junk that seem to accumulate when you live in the country on 5 acres of land.

Planting new flowerbeds, then weeding and protecting them from hungry deer was an ongoing yet enjoyable task. Hosting a wedding in our yard spurred us to previously unknown pinnacles of cleaning, de-cluttering and fixing every sagging fence, collapsed shed and eyesore that we had blissfully ignored for a decade or more.

Luckily, we had a small army of our combined families and friends helping to make the wedding a memorable day. I stopped to take a deep breath while I looked around at everyone present from all over the United States; Katie's mom and sisters plus Tucker's grandmas and grandpas, aunts and uncles, cousins and lifelong friends busily working together on this one beautiful spot.

I thought about how each person, in their own amazing way had contributed to my son's healing and commitment to a better life for himself. They had also supported me; often just listening from miles away as I cried while pouring out my hopes, fears, and uncertainties concerning Tucker's health and the SCD program. Again and again, month after month, they listened and reassured me. Whenever they had flown in for a visit I had looked to them for much needed help with the constant cooking chores.

Thinking of all this, I glanced up at my friend Donna, who had driven up from Oregon a week ago to help with wedding preparations. She was sweating in the hot sun while assisting others in creating a gravel edged cedar chip pathway for the married couple to walk down tomorrow. A year ago she had come for a visit

133

after a sad divorce, sharing her sorrow while helping me harvest vegetables from our garden. We washed, chopped and processed them into thirty-quart jars of SCD vegetable soup for Tucker. I took advantage of an extra pair of hands whenever they appeared.

I scanned the yard once more, stopping to rest my eyes on the familiar faces of my husband Steve and son Dylan teasing each other as they lifted one end of the heavy wedding tent in unison. I felt a tremendous gratitude for their generosity in taking a step back during the two years following Tucker's diagnosis and slow path to healing. It's not easy having a wife or mother on the brink of desperation, focusing elsewhere for long periods of time; but they helped keep my worst fears at bay and reminded me that laughter and joy always had a spot in our home no matter what we were facing.

Tucker and Katie appeared near the tent, arm in arm, shared smiles of anticipation on their faces, love in their hearts for everyone present. They had brought such joy to each other's lives I thought as I watched them run over to grab a corner pole, helping to secure the tent as the stakes were pounded in one by one. A promise of a shared life filled with laughter, love, and gratitude would be celebrated by all tomorrow at their wedding.

The much anticipated day finally arrived and everything was beautiful. I had been a little worried over the past week about Tucker handling the typical wedding stress without going into a flare up but he remained calm and collected. When the musicians began playing Pachelbel's Canon and Katie accompanied by her mother came into full view my heart was bursting with happiness. Tucker was waiting for her; standing with his grandfather Paul (who performed the ceremony), his brother Dylan, and his best man Kale. Three years ago I had wondered if Tucker would ever enjoy a "normal" life. I should have known he would pull off not only a normal life but also an active and rich one filled with all the things he loved. These days of joyous celebration for the future of Tucker and Katie were gifts born on the wings of perseverance through unforeseen setbacks and lessons in hope. Diligently following the SCD plan for over three years had healed my son from the inside out and it showed. Tucker radiated vigorous health and his boyish good looks were back. He actually looked more like an eighteen-year-old twin to his brother Dylan than a twenty-seven year old married man.

The SCD lifestyle is literally stress free for Tucker now. Katie eats the same foods for their dinners together but supplements with wheat bread sandwiches, Greek style yogurt and her own homemade desserts for work lunches. She enjoys ginger snaps, pumpkin muffins and carrot cake desserts. These treats have never appealed to Tucker and he makes his own cookies and cakes using almond flour. In the end it works for them.

My son has become quite the gourmet cook and now gives me advice about preparing meats and vegetables in new ways. We are now kale chip and winter squash fries aficionados. We also learned to eat more salads when Tucker lived with us and we continue to enjoy them daily. My husband watched Tucker slice and eat an apple with peanut butter every night and now frequently enjoys one with thin slices of sharp cheddar cheese.

I struggled daily (and still do!) with taming my sweet tooth and stood in awe at Tuckers ability to do so. When the whole extended family gathers for holidays we eat SCD meals with non-SCD side dishes. Tucker picks and chooses foods that are legal for him and we've learned it's easy to tweak almost any recipe to accommodate the SCD requirements.

I still help supplement his diet by canning vegetable soup for quick meals, freezing spaghetti sauce made from our homegrown tomatoes (we also grow the spaghetti squash,) plus I make SCD legal jam and pesto. Our garden is always overflowing with surplus vegetables so I have lots of experience dealing with excess beans, raspberries, peppers, tomatoes and of course zucchini. We usually have venison or elk in the freezer so jerky is a regular snack we prepare in our dehydrator for all to share. I have fun experimenting with canning ketchup or barbeque sauce and am always on the lookout for new SCD recipes.

I strongly recommend planting at least a small salad garden and regularly shopping at your local farmers market. Many small market gardeners can deliver boxes of fresh produce to you on a weekly basis through a CSA (Community Sponsored Agriculture) Program. This will encourage you to try different vegetables and you may find a new favorite. I never cared too much for winter squash but now I can't live without it. We store over forty butternuts, sweet mamas, and spaghetti squashes to last us through the winter and enjoy them on a regular basis. Flower beds can be transformed into beautiful lettuce, pepper and tomato gardens or backyards dug up to accommodate full size gardens. I did just that when I was thirteen years old and my parents went away for the weekend. They returned to their entire backyard of grass quietly composting in black plastic garbage bags and hand tilled soil neatly planted with rows of seeds. I even had the little seed packets stapled to stakes at the end of each row announcing what vegetables would soon be bursting forth from each straight line of black soil. My parents were finally happy a couple months later when we were eating bushels of fresh produce.

Cooking from scratch using fresh ingredients can be a fun and entertaining routine for the whole family to enjoy. My husband likes to sit out of the way snapping beans or chopping vegetables while everyone else is bumping into each other preparing their own special dish to share at dinner. Tucker and I continue to phone each other frequently to share delicious recipes or special concoctions we have invented. If you approach preparing meals as a pleasurable venture then it will become just that.

The Specific Carbohydrate Diet works. It just does. You have to be vigilant with eating only legal foods, sometimes even evaluating and eliminating those legal foods that don't settle well. You should experiment using your gut as your guide; if a certain food gives you heartburn, gas or diarrhea, eliminate it for a couple weeks before trying that food again. If uncomfortable symptoms persist then leave it off your menu for a year. Tucker found he could not tolerate a soup made with roasted eggplant but could enjoy small eggplant slices grilled crisply. The diet seems to be a give and take formula with some food preparations being OK and others producing problems. Again, use your judgment and listen to your body.

The SCD definitely takes planning and effort in the beginning but quickly becomes a way of life. Commit to embracing it one hundred percent for a month. Evaluate how you feel on the diet and continue on from there. It's easier if you think of IBD as an allergic response to starches. If you had breathing problems and itchy rashes after eating dairy products would you continue consuming them despite your discomfort? It's the same way with an IBD. The colon can't process starches. It first reacts with gas, bloating, diarrhea and pain and can escalate to severe pain, bloody diarrhea, weight loss, and possibly a stay in the hospital.

Ask yourself which sounds harder to do: regain good health and energy to participate in the things you love to do by spending extra time in the kitchen or enduring poor health while chained to the toilet, swallowing lots of expensive pills with risky side-effects but eating whatever you want?

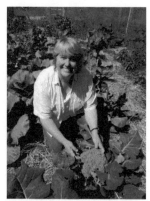

Mom in her Idaho garden

After a few bumps in the road the answer became crystal clear to Tucker; he chose health and living an active life with the SCD. If you falter with the diet get right back on it one hundred percent, eventually it will become your way of living life and you too will enjoy good health.

It was truly an honor and privilege to play a role in my son's healing. I had felt so overwhelmed and inadequate when he was first diagnosed with ulcerated colitis. I have since discovered a power within me I didn't know I had. When you keep saying tomorrow will be a better day eventually you start to believe it, and then in small ways it does become a better day. Gratitude built in my heart for my family and friends. I realized we weren't alone in our daily struggles and I felt stronger knowing that. I witnessed raw courage watching Tucker break through challenges and learn gratitude for the daily, small pleasures of life.

We wrote this book to ease your struggles with IBD. We wrote the kind of book we were desperate to read when Tucker was first diagnosed.

May you find peace and healing in all that life offers up and hope with every new day.

Chapter 14

~Balance~

So here I am, writing this story in my house in Boise. It's almost the new year of 2011 and when I think back on all the struggles, triumphs, and lessons I have learned over the years, I am at a loss for words.

I recently completed my student teaching experience—my capstone assignment and am one semester away from earning my teaching degree.

I remain in good health, and my commitment to the SCD way of life is still strong. I experienced a flare-up last fall; right before starting my student teaching and in my mind this was brought about by the added stress. I managed to complete the experience and recover fully, yet it remains a vivid memory that UC is lying in wait.

I have definitely become more adjusted to the rollercoaster of my life, and the adventures it takes me on. In one sense I feel grateful for the lessons that UC has taught me, yet in another sense I would like to forget many of the memories that come up. It's a trade off, I guess.

Old memories were brought back to life last summer when my dad learned he also has UC. Months of bloody diarrhea, weight loss, and fatigue brought us all to wonder if he had colon cancer or an E.coli infection since he was past the age when most people get UC. He had no previous indicators of UC in his adolescence or twenties. Plus, what a weird coincidence for both of us to have it, even knowing that there is a genetic factor with IBD.

I jumped into the helping mode and gave him all of the information I could about my experience. After two months of suffering and a weight loss worse than mine, he was officially diagnosed with UC. He, along with the help of his wife Jodi, promptly started the SCD and began a round of

Prednisone. Within a month he was off Prednisone and committed fully to the SCD way of life and in good health.

To this day, he has made a remarkable recovery. He has even been able to have the occasional illegal food and not suffer the consequences of a relapse. UC is unique to each person and you will have to find what works for you.

Having UC and eating SCD brought my dad and I closer. A unique bond developed between us that came from our shared experience of hardship, disciplined diet, and a hope that we could heal ourselves from the inside out.

Even though it was extremely frightening and difficult to witness the destruction of the disease upon someone you love, it was equally satisfying to set into action the blueprint I had meticulously followed throughout the years. The diet, the yogurt maker, chicken soup, the dos and don'ts. I, along with others like my mom and his wife Jodi, quickly went into action and set about teaching him the healing process from the beginning. The learning curve was shorter for him because of all we had learned. By writing this book I hope to do the same for you.

My life today has a good balance. I am no longer a victim of UC. If I do experience an occasional relapse, I know that I will get through it and become stronger from it. I have found a routine with the SCD and this makes things easier. My typical day starts with a bowl of yogurt with frozen blueberries, honey, and a handful of crushed walnuts. I usually have some sort of tea like green, herbal, or yerba mate. For lunch, I usually have either last night's dinner leftovers or I make a grilled cheese, tuna, or peanut butter and jelly sandwich using bread from a modified Lois Lang recipe from BTVC.

Dinners are a revolving door of new and old ideas but with some weekly standards thrown in. We make nachos almost every week, which consists of making chips with a modified John's pizza recipe #2 out of the BTVC and topping the chips with cheese, onions, diced green peppers, and olives. With that we have sides of legal refried black beans, homemade guacamole, and salsa. Other dinners that have become standard weekly affairs are Thai coconut soup and taco bowls, which can all be found in the resource section of this book. For dessert, I usually have yogurt, or whip up a cookie recipe or apple slices with peanut butter.

My alcoholic drink of choice is red wine and my gut seems to tolerate this much more than some of the legal hard liquors like gin or vodka. Given this, I usually don't drink the very refreshing gin and tonic (using diet tonic and fresh limes) very often. Diet sodas are an interesting treat about once every two-three months but I would caution you to be very careful with them as I notice gut changes the moment I drink one. Like I said earlier in the book also be very careful of the peanut butter caramel recipe that is out and about in SCD cookbooks, and for that matter be careful of any legal desserts that are caramel in consistency and contain more caramel than they do nuts. I do fine with the caramel nut-balls but not the peanut butter caramels or peanut brittle type desserts which led to a flare up.

Having a garden is also a great way to not only get good quality produce at cheap prices it also allows you to formulate food plans more easily. For example, if you have lots of spinach, you make something that has spinach in it. If you have lettuce coming out your ears, you make huge salads for lunch and dinner. Having a garden also helps you to learn about the food you eat.

Supplements are a touchy subject to many. You will be hard pressed to find anyone who is dealing with a disease who does not have some sort of supplement plan in place. There are many supplements so I will just let you know what I take. Currently I take probiotics (SCD legal variety) twice a day and folic acid once a day. That's it. I used to take a multi vitamin but realized my diet was probably supplying all the nutrients I needed on a daily basis. The probiotics I feel are a real help for my condition and can sometimes stop an advancing flare up. The probiotics function to increase healthy bacteria like acidophilus in your intestinal tract and have been shown in many research studies to be of benefit, especially to IBD patients. If I had one supplement to recommend, probiotics would be it.

B-vitamins and folic acid are a class of vitamins many with IBD are deficient in, due to malabsorption issues. I felt no ill effects from taking a B-complex vitamin, yet I felt I just did not need it and that I could obtain plenty of B-vitamins from meats and other foods. Folic acid is my insurance plan for this class of vitamins and so far it has covered me.

Other things that I have researched and have tried but have either stopped taking or take on an irregular basis are listed here: Curcumin (anti-inflammatory), oil of oregano (anti-bacterial), multi vitamins (overall health), B-complex (increasing impaired B-vitamin levels), plant sterinols (anti-inflammatory), L-Glutamine (a source of fuel for cells lining the intestines), Vitamin D (promotes calcium absorption in the gut and body), and activated charcoal (emergency decontaminant in the gastrointestinal tract). None of these supplements caused my symptoms to get worse but I cannot say that any of them for sure helped in a profound way. It was hard to tell while being on other treatments, i.e. medications, SCD, probiotics, etc. Some of the more interesting and obscure treatments that I have heard of but have not tried are listed here: THC oil, fecal transplants (human probiotics infusions), cats claw, colloidal silver, Helminthic worm therapy, probiotics enemas, and Vitamin E enemas. The supplement part of UC is an area that each person needs to research and study for themselves.

After suffering for years with low back and hip pain, some of which I attribute to UC, I finally went to a physical therapist for help. He gave me a whole series of core strengthening techniques along with a stretching routine.

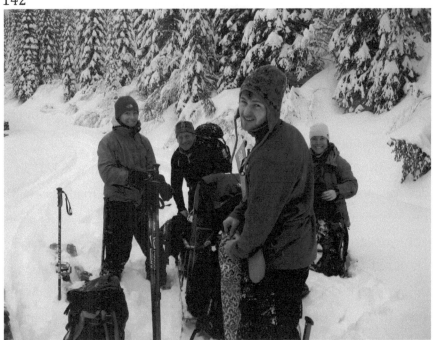

Skiing! Katie, Joe, Dylan, and Jodi

I have tried massage therapists, chiropractors, naprapaths, and orthopedic doctors to experience temporary relief but I can tell you physical therapy is the way to go. Not only did it diminish much of the pain I usually experience but it is also something I can do on my own, and not have to pay for over and over again.

Another part of my life that I have really had to pay attention to is stress. Most everyone that has some sort of bowel issue will tell you that stress can wreak havoc on your digestive system. Even from a young age I can remember the feeling of holding my stress in my stomach. I would always feel nauseous in stressful situations and my stomach would get rock hard under pressing conditions. This was not good, then or now. I remember, as a teenager thinking that stress and the way it felt in my gut, would someday give me cancer. Well, it didn't give me cancer but it may have given me UC.

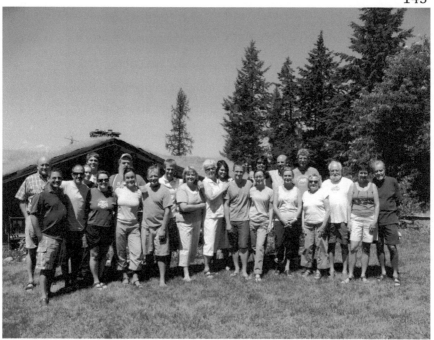

Family and friends after the wedding

My dad has given me many good pieces of advice but one that really stuck in my mind was this: Breath in the things you want, and breath out the things you don't. This mantra has become essential to me when confronted with stressful situations. It works for me. I also love to exercise and be outdoors in the fresh air. This for me reduces the stress and thoughts of worry that tend to creep into my mind. It helps me focus on the essentials and forget the rest. Who needs it!

In the kitchen, Katie and I have begun to branch out into different ethnic food groups. Converting recipes to SCD legal has become easier to do with substitutions for various ingredients. Dealing with the SCD is no longer a chore but a fact of life. I figure it out like a puzzle. Substitute almond flour for wheat in a recipe; exchange baking powder with baking soda.

Cooking good quality food brings out something basic and nourishing to my soul; the cutting and slicing of the vegetables, the way meat reacts with the addition of garlic to produce a sizzle and a sensual smell.

Sometimes when I'm really in the groove of cooking a good meal, music in the background and glass of wine to the side, I feel a very strong purpose in what I'm doing. No longer is it just ingredients but rather a creative combination that gives health and nourishment to my life.

Even if you don't know it yet, you do have the skills in your own two hands to create a better life for yourself. Use them to create the food you need and to open the doors to the way of life you deserve and desire. Put the demons of the past behind you and focus on the realities of today. Think of your disease as less of a disorder or abnormality and more like a characteristic that requires different needs.

Ulcerative colitis has taught me that we all have something to deal with. How one chooses to deal with a crisis defines us. Will you let your disease define you or will you define yourself through the things that love and inspire you? I cooked, studied, failed, and triumphed but I never lost sight of who I am and who I want to be. I am inspired by mountains and sheer rock walls rising from the ground. I am inspired by the generosity and love of those around me. Now too, I enjoy sharing my passion for life while talking to others about the SCD. I feel the love of others when I spend time with them living life. For a time, I didn't do these things because I was sick. I was consumed with fear of the future and was waiting, instead of living.

The SCD gave me not only the strength to move forward with my life but also the ability to be involved in the healing process. I needed to change the way I thought and add new ways to reach my goals. Who cares if I had to climb a mountain with a pad in my pants? I was going to do it and I did! If you wait around for things to happen, just be prepared to wait a while. My journey contained many ups and downs but I never bought the idea that this was as good as it was going to get. No thanks. I wanted better and I went out and found it.

~Two steps forward, one step back~

Standard Food Recipes

Biscuits

Making this versatile bread recipe has become a monthly affair. I use it for sandwiches, toast in the morning, grilled cheeses, etc. I usually make two batches, one after the other to have enough for a couple weeks, and to use up the amount of dry curd cottage cheese that comes in the packages I am able to buy. The biscuits freeze well and can be pulled out as needed. Adapted from Lois Lang recipe in *Breaking The Vicious Cycle*.

3 ½ cups almond flour

2 tablespoons melted butter

1 cup dry curd cottage cheese or 1 cup dripped yogurt

1 teaspoon baking soda

¼ teaspoon salt

2 eggs

1 tablespoon spices, such as: caraway seeds, Italian spice, etc. (optional)

Mix the butter, dry curd cottage cheese, baking soda, salt, eggs, and any spices in a food processor until thick (about 30sec). Add the almond flour and mix until fully combined. Consistency should be that of very thick cookie batter and should be very sticky.

Form dough into about 3" diameter disks with water-wet hands and place on an oiled baking sheet or parchment paper.

Bake at 350 degrees for 25-30 min. Let cool completely before cutting.

Pizza and chip dough

This is a great dough recipe adapted/modified from John's pizza recipe #2 in *Breaking The Vicious Cycle*. I usually double or triple the recipe and keep the formed extra dough balls in the freezer for quick use.

<u>Dough:</u>

1 cup almond flour

1 egg

1 teaspoon olive oil

¼ teaspoon salt

1 teaspoon Italian spices (optional)

Mix everything together until fully combined. Form into small fist sized balls and wrap with cling wrap for storage in the refrigerator or freezer.

Pizza:

Roll dough out onto a baking sheet covered with parchment paper or onto a nonstick surface. Roll out dough by placing the cling wrap over the dough as you roll it to prevent dough from sticking to the roller. Remove cling wrap and bake dough for about 10-15 minutes until lightly brown. Add homemade tomato sauce or pesto, then add any SCD legal toppings you'd like (mushrooms, peppers, olives, spinach, chard, onions, chicken).

Top with cheese and bake for about 30 minutes at 350 degrees. *For a tougher crust that does not get soggy, add cheddar or Parmesan cheese to the crust before adding the sauce and bake until brown. You can also experiment with different crust thicknesses to see which one you like the best.

Chips:

Roll out dough as in the pizza recipe. Using a knife, cut dough into chip-sized squares like a checkerboard.

Bake at 350 degrees for 10-15 minutes or until lightly brown. Use for dips, nachos or cheese and crackers.

Burrito Wraps

What a revelation to have a wrap to hold food ingredients. I often thought to myself "I don't care what the heck it tastes like I just want something to <u>hold</u> my food" Eating burrito fillings plain and in a bowl gets old and sometimes is not practical while in the backcountry. These wraps are tough, flexible, and easy to make. The perfect triple combo!

*Makes about 4-8 wraps depending on size

5 eggs

½ cup almond flour

1 teaspoon honey

1/8 teaspoon salt

Olive oil for frying

Whisk all ingredients together making sure no lumps exist. Heat a lightly oiled, non-stick; flat pan till it is hot (add a few drops water or batter and make sure it sizzles on contact). Add 1/4-1/2 cup batter to the pan. Upon adding batter quickly lift and turn pan in a circular motion to thin out the batter and create a large round burrito shape.

Cook for about 20-30 seconds or until wrap has a slight sheen. Carefully lift edges and flip. Repeat a few times until wrap is lightly browned or to your desired specifications. Remove to a plate with paper towels and let cool. Store in the refrigerator, freezer or cooler.

Thai Coconut Soup

I really love this soup and it has become a weekly affair in our house. It's rich, creamy, healthy, and tastes great! Make sure all of your ingredients are SCD legal. Call the manufacturers if you are not sure.

1 tablespoon peanut butter

1 tablespoon olive oil

1 medium sized chicken breast cut into small pieces

1-2 large leeks cut into 2" matchsticks

32 fluid ounces chicken broth

2 (15 ounce) cans of unsweetened coconut milk

1 tablespoon lime zest

¼ cup lime juice (about 2 limes)

1 small bunch cilantro

Couple shakes of cayenne pepper (optional)

Mix together the oil and peanut butter into a watery paste in the pan. Add the chicken chunks and sauté over medium heat until chicken is cooked. Remove the chicken to another plate trying to reserve as much oil in the pan as possible. To the pan add the leeks and cook until soft and translucent (add more oil if needed).

Once the leeks are cooked, add stock, coconut milk, and lime zest. Bring to a simmer. Return the chicken to the pot, add the lime juice, cayenne, and cilantro. Serve immediately and do not let the soup boil.

Nachos

This is a great meal when you feel like having something that is not SCD legal, yet it is! I probably make this dish every week and I never seem to get tired of it.

<u>Chips:</u>

1 chip/pizza dough portion made into chips (P.147 & 148)

<u>Toppings:</u> **(use however much you want)**

Cheddar cheese

Diced green chilies

Black olives

Onion (diced)

<u>Sides:</u>

Refried black beans (SCD) and guacamole

Place the cooked chips into a pie pan and add the toppings on top. It is best to start with the cheese then go down the list. Bake for 20-30 minutes at 350 degrees.

To make the refried black beans soak black beans overnight (empty and exchange water once or twice) then cook until soft. Mash softened beans with salt and olive oil to taste

For guacamole cut two ripe avocados and place in a bowl. Add a tablespoon of finely chopped onion and cilantro, the juice of half a lime and salt to taste. Mash and mix to your desired consistency.

Jerky

Jerky is a great snack in so many ways. It doesn't go rancid very quickly; it stores and packs well, its light and tastes great, and its full of protein. I eat this around the house and while on outdoor adventures. A handful of jerky stuffed in a pocket makes a long climb that much easier and tasty! You need a dehydrator for this.

Lean round steak or roast (beef, elk, venison)

½-1 teaspoon salt per pound of meat

Pepper to taste (around 1/8 teaspoon per pound)

Remove any fat and slice meat into 1/8-inch thick strips and add to a large bowl. Season each layer of meat with the salt and pepper (add any other spices you'd like) and mix everything together. Let the meat mixture sit in the refrigerator for twelve hours (or overnight) to marinate. It can marinate for longer – a day or two if it's kept refrigerated. Once marinated, lay the strips of meat in a single layer on the dehydrator racks and set the machine to the manufacturers meat setting. Check after 8-10 hours. Remove the meat when it is dry and slightly hard. Taste test for your personal preference. The drier it is the longer it keeps.

Butternut Squash Fries

Butternut squash is a very tasty and versatile food. I mash it to make mock mashed potatoes or sauté it cubed and lightly tossed with olive oil, a pinch of crushed dried chili peppers, a little rosemary, and salt to taste. This makes an elegant side dish and comfort food. But my favorite thing to do with butternut squash is to make squash fries. This dish will definitely "squash" your cravings for starchy food!

1 medium sized butternut squash (*optional: Use carrots instead)

Olive oil

Salt

Spices (garlic, chili powder, oregano, paprika, etc.)

Use a vegetable peeler to peel the butternut squash, then cut in half and scrape out the seeds and fibers. Next slice and cut the squash into either French fry sized pieces or cubes and place on a large cookie sheet with sides on it. Toss the squash pieces with a Tablespoon or two of olive oil (just enough to coat). Add a dusting of salt and spices and continue to toss. Bake at 400 degrees for about 40 minutes or until the squash pieces are just beginning to become crisp. Periodically toss and flip the mixture to assure both sides of the squash are being cooked. Sometimes, I mix up a *yogurt sauce* using yogurt, salt, and spices like cumin and chili powder. It's a delicious dipping sauce for the fries.

Peanut Butter Cookies

These cookies are a nice, filling snack that tends to hold up well while travelling. Feel free to increase or decrease the amount of honey to suit your palette. I like them with just a hint of sweetness, which also seems to be easier on my stomach.

2 cups almond flour

¼ teaspoon baking soda

1/8 teaspoon ground cinnamon

½ cup chopped walnuts

2 eggs

1 teaspoon pure vanilla -SCD legal variety

½ cup honey (more or less)

1 cup unsweetened peanut butter

2 tablespoons melted butter

Mix together the almond flour, baking soda, cinnamon, and walnuts. Next, add the eggs, vanilla, honey, peanut butter, and melted butter. Mix well, then using a large spoon drop heaping tablespoons onto a greased baking sheet.

Bake at 325 degrees for 20-30 minutes or until cookies are just starting to brown.

Homemade Yogurt

This is the standard yogurt that I make just about every week. I choose whole milk because I like a full fat, thick yogurt. This is not to say that you can't use 2% milk if you would like to cut out more fat in your diet. The only two yogurt starters that I have used have come from either Lucy's Kitchen shop or from GI Pro Health. Both make a delicious yogurt and have a proven track record.

1 half-gallon whole or 2% milk

Yogurt starter

Place milk in large saucepan over medium high heat. Stir constantly until milk just comes to a boil. Remove from heat and cool (I place the pan in the sink with cold water surrounding pot). Cool until the recommended temperature for your yogurt starter. Pour a cup of the cooled milk into your yogurt container-add starter (amounts will vary by brand) and mix together thoroughly. Add the remaining milk to the container and gently stir. Follow directions for your yogurt maker with the exception that you must ferment the yogurt for at least 24 hours but no more than 30 hours.

Check to see that your yogurt maker does not heat the yogurt more than 115 degrees, which could kill the fermenting bacteria. If your yogurt maker does run hot you can try and remove the lid or purchase a dimmer switch to lower the heating temperature.

Once the yogurt has fermented for 24 hours, remove container from yogurt maker and refrigerate for 6-8 hours to cease fermentation.

Favorites

Fried Cheese

This is a great one-ingredient snack when you want something that is crunchy, salty, and rich. Similar to the flavor of snack cheese crackers, yet without all of the illegal ingredients.

Sliced medium cheddar cheese

Slice the cheddar cheese into 1/8 inch slices and place onto heated non-stick pan over medium heat. After a couple minutes of sizzling, the cheese should start to thin out and get air holes in it as the oil separates. Do not attempt to turn until edges are light brown and crispy. The cheese should not stick to your spatula while attempting to flip. When the cheese is lightly browned use a spatula to flip it over and cook the other side. The second side tends to brown very quickly. Once browned on both sides, remove to paper towel to remove excess oil. Let cool to become crispy. Practice makes perfect on this recipe!

Roasted Nuts

These are a salty snack, and a good alternative to the nut mixes you can buy. They make great travel food and are packed with good nutrients. We like the nuts with just salt but feel free to add various spices like garlic powder, chili powder or curry. Also, different nut varieties can be used to suit your taste.

Melt 1 Tablespoon butter in medium bowl.

Add 2 cups pecans (or other nut variety).

Stir well to coat nuts with butter.

Spread on a cookie sheet with sides.

Sprinkle with salt. Add other spices if desired…

Bake at 350 degrees for 5 minutes.

Remove from oven and cool in pan.

Enjoy!

Candied Nuts

Feeling like something sweet, salty, and crunchy? These nuts are a nice treat to keep around the house or in a bag for travels. They also make a nice snack for the Christmas holidays. Adapted from *Breaking The Vicious Cycle*.

1 pound raw nuts (almonds, walnuts, pecans, pumpkin seeds)

2 egg whites

½ cup honey

¼ cup butter

1/8 teaspoon salt

½ teaspoon cinnamon

Toast nuts on a baking sheet at 300 degrees for ten minutes.

Remove pan from oven and let cool.

Beat egg whites till soft peaks form.

Add salt and cinnamon then drizzle in honey while continuing to beat egg whites.

Fold nuts into the egg white mixture.

Add butter to pan and place pan in oven until butter is melted.

Add the egg white/nut mixture to the buttered pan and spread to a single layer stirring the butter into the nuts.

Bake for 30-40 minutes at 300 degrees stirring nut mixture every 10 minutes to incorporate the butter into the nuts.

Remove pan from oven. Let cool 10 minutes in pan then remove to a bowl so that the nuts don't stick to the pan. As the nuts cool break them apart so they don't form a huge glob.

Store in a closed container at room temperature or in the refrigerator for longer periods.

Caramel Nut Balls

A family favorite whether you follow the SCD or not. A real treat that puts your sweet tooth back in its place. These make great high-energy snacks for adventurous pursuits, except that in cold environments they can become very hard. Pecans and almonds can be substituted for walnuts if desired. Adapted from Lucy's Cookbook.

1 cup honey

4 tablespoons butter

¼ teaspoon salt

3 teaspoons vanilla

3 cups coarsely chopped walnuts

1½ cups finely chopped walnuts

Bring honey, butter, and salt to a foamy boil, lower heat and continue to simmer (it will be foamy and bubbly) for 15 minutes. Stir in the 3 cups chopped walnuts and continue simmering for another 5 minutes stirring frequently. Remove from heat, add vanilla, and stir well. Allow mixture to cool enough to handle with bare hands (about 15 minutes). Spread finely chopped walnuts onto a large plate or baking dish.

Roll caramel nut mixture into 1 inch round balls using your hands, then roll in the finely chopped walnuts to coat.

Layer with wax paper in a sealed container and leave at room temperature or in the refrigerator.

Huckleberry Ice Cream

Having ice cream on a hot summer day can be true paradise. Invest in an ice cream maker such as a *Donvier*^{TM} *Sorbetiere*, available at Lucy's Kitchen Shop or other online retailers. The ice cream maker is super easy to use and can produce great frozen desserts in around 15 minutes. To make this dessert taste even better go pick the huckleberries or blueberries yourself!

Place all ingredients into a large blender and blend:

1 (14oz) can SCD legal coconut milk

14oz (use empty coconut milk can to measure) yogurt

1 cup frozen huckleberries or blueberries

1/4 – 1/2 cup honey (I like to use only 1/4 cup)

1 tablespoon vanilla

Blend all ingredients then pour mixture into the pre-frozen ice cream maker. Follow manufactures directions. Leftovers can be placed in Tupperware then into the freezer. After freezing the ice cream will need to be left out for 20-30 minutes prior to eating or placed in the microwave for 15-20 seconds to become soft enough to eat.

Blueberry Muffins

This makes a nice firm muffin that resembles a white flour muffin you would buy at a bakery. It's the perfect treat to put a pat of butter on for breakfast or a mid-day snack. Sometimes I also mash a very ripe banana into the mix for a different flavor. Makes about 12 muffins.

2½ cups almond flour

½ teaspoon baking soda

1/8 teaspoon salt

¼ cup melted butter

¼-½ cup honey (more or less as desired)

3 eggs

¼ cup SCD yogurt

¾ cup blueberries (small and frozen blueberries work best)

Mix together the first three ingredients.

Add everything else except for the blueberries and mix well with a whisk.

Add blueberries to the batter and mix to combine.

Spoon batter into paper muffin cups and fill about ¾ full.

Bake at 325 degrees for 30 minutes or until toothpick inserted comes out clean.

Kale Chips

Unique, nutritious, and a fun chip substitute. A great way to utilize kale from your garden or make a fun snack for your family or guests. Kids love these!

1 bunch curly leafed kale (approximately 20 leaves or how ever much you want).

Olive oil

Salt or other seasoning

Wash kale and remove large portion of the stems. Let dry thoroughly.

Place kale on ungreased baking sheet and brush both sides of leaves very lightly with olive oil. Lightly season with salt or another legal seasoning of your choice.

Place into a 350-degree oven and watch very closely so they do not burn. Usually they take about 10 minutes to crisp up and at this point they are done. Remove pan from oven and place kale on paper towels to absorb any excess oil.

Homemade SCD Jam or Jelly

We have not come across a jam or jelly product made without pectin so I came up with this version. It's sweetened with honey and tastes great on SCD biscuits and muffins or stirred into yogurt. Can also be used to make jam filled cookies.

Put a couple cups of fruit (I've tried raspberries and huckleberries with excellent results, peaches would be good too) in a saucepan over medium heat and mash the fruit as it starts to heat.

Add honey to taste, start with ¼ cup or so....

Continue stirring constantly until fruit is reduced in volume by about half and has thickened. Remove from heat and it will thicken as it cools.

If it is too runny for a PBJ sandwich then next time reduce the volume a little more, the runnier product is easier to stir into yogurt.

Cooking for a Week

Here are my ideas for making a week's worth of meals in one afternoon for two people or one hungry young man on steroids. I found it was easier to set aside a three to four hour block of time to pre-plan and get the bulk of my cooking done for the week ahead.

Getting your weekly muffin and cookie baking done in one afternoon means you will have those staples on hand when the munchies hit after work or school. In the same afternoon, you can roast a chicken, bake a simple crust-less quiche and meatloaf, and assemble a large salad. It sounds like a lot of work but the trick is to have all your ingredients out, reuse the bowl you mixed your quiche eggs in for the muffin batter (no need to wash it) then use again without rinsing for the cookie dough, after that a quick rinse and wipe with a paper towel before throwing your meatloaf ingredients in that same bowl.

Be an efficient cook and by all means have fun. Turn on some music, pour yourself a glass of wine and put some love into your food. Creating meals can be an artistic pursuit instead of drudgery. A relaxing hobby not a chore.

Each day then requires just a couple quick embellishments (like melting a piece of cheese on a slice of meat loaf and quickly steaming some green beans) to your preassembled main dish and you have a nourishing meal in a couple of minutes after a long day.

This is a sample menu for one week of meals and can be modified to suit your tastes and needs. Amounts are for one or two people. Switch the chicken or pork roast for a nice filet of salmon one night but be sure to cook fish the night it is to be eaten.

The idea is to have two or three main dishes prepared ahead of time, along with plenty of snacks on hand for when you are too tired to cook or need to eat something RIGHT NOW! Following the diet 100% depends heavily upon being prepared because it's easier to resist eating illegal foods if you have a lot of SCD options.

Written below you will find an ingredient list with explanations of some foods added on. As you compile your grocery list for the week feel free to substitute anything such as, cauliflower for broccoli or salmon for a meatloaf. I am simply showing you what a basic weekly meal plan looked like while I was cooking for Tucker. We played around with more gourmet options when we had the time and the SCD got easier. I would strongly recommend starting with the basics and adding more options, as it becomes a lifestyle not an event.

Ingredient list:

SCD yogurt- needs to be started 24 hours prior.

Almond flour- buy this in bulk from the internet- Lucy's kitchen Shop and Honeyville Food Products have good sources.

SCD legal vanilla- you can buy online with no sugar or glycerin added. I make my own using a cup of vodka with a couple vanilla beans split and soaked in the vodka. Use a tall thin bottle so the beans are submerged or cut them in half and leave them in the vodka, it will get stronger as you use it, takes about 2 weeks to build up any strength.

1 gallon or half gallon milk- for yogurt whole milk is the best

1 box yogurt starter- *Yogourmet*[TM] and *GI Prostart*[TM] are brands we have used with success.

1 dozen eggs

Salad ingredients (lettuce, celery, carrots, whatever else you enjoy plus extras amounts for chicken soup)

1 head broccoli or cauliflower (both if you like to eat steamed veggies with your dinners)

1 zucchini (for meatloaf)

1 -4oz can green chilies for a chili rellenos style quiche

Onions (nice to have around if you like them in your meals)

1 head garlic- if you like it

Fresh fruits-1 lemon, 5 apples, 5 oranges, 1 fresh pineapple (if you like to snack on it and have it in smoothies), one bunch ripe bananas (I usually buy the discounted bag of ripe ones then peel and cut some up and freeze them in a freezer bag to use in smoothies)

A bag of frozen blueberries– at least 4 cups worth, keep frozen

2 pounds of hamburger

1 whole chicken

1 package Chicken sausages- check labels for sugar-there are many varieties, some made with apples and gouda or sweet red pepper and garlic that are like a gourmet smokie/hot dog but do not contain sugar –We buy ours at Costco but I'm sure they are everywhere.

1 bag or glass jar of fresh (not in a tin can) sauerkraut

Olive oil

White wine vinegar

Mustard (SCD legal stone-ground type)

Mayonnaise- made with honey not sugar, you can find this in your health food store or make your own.

1 large butternut squash

1 pound butter

1 bag frozen green beans

2 lb block of Cheddar cheese

8 oz Monterey jack cheese

Swiss cheese– at least 8 ounces, for the quiche

Gouda, Jarlsberg, Gorgonzola, or any other aged cheeses if you enjoy a small cheese, fruit, and walnut platter after dinner for dessert. Fresh grapes and a nice glass of wine pair nicely with this arrangement.

Apple, orange, or grape juice- (preferably fresh squeezed and not from concentrate) or other juice you enjoy- no sugar added, you will use these for smoothies. Regular Welch's™ grape juice is SCD verified.

Nuts (Walnuts, Almonds, Pecans, Cashews, Peanuts)- you might as well buy them in 2-5 lb quantities, as you will use a lot of them in this diet. They store well in the refrigerator or freezer if you buy them in bulk.

Almond butter or peanut butter- if tolerated

Honey- buy at least a quart, it stores well in the cupboard and you use it a lot

1 lb unsweetened dried coconut- get it at any health food store- keeps well on the shelf

Raisins- we will only use about ½ cup but they store well and you will use them in other recipes or for snacking

Dates- unsweetened, Medjool are the best in our opinion. We only need four dates for this week but they store for many months so get extra if you want.

Cinnamon, poultry seasoning, baking soda, salt and pepper are probably already in your cupboard

Quart size freezer bags are nice to have around; you can put a couple slices of meatloaf in one to freeze for another week if you can't finish a whole one in a few days.

1. Make **chicken stock** if you bought a whole chicken-use the chicken backs and neck, put in soup pot, cover with 4 cups water, add a bay leaf or two, 1 tsp basil, 1 tsp oregano, 1 tsp poultry seasoning, a couple slices onion and the leafy parts of your celery. Allow to simmer for 2 hours. Strain broth, save meat from bones. Add ½ cup chopped onions, 1 cup chopped celery, 1 cup carrot slices, 1 cup green beans, and reserved meat to broth. Simmer 30 minutes. Salt and pepper to taste. Cool slightly then refrigerate.

2. Preheat oven to 325 degrees, then assemble the **blueberry muffin** recipe: See page 163 and bake for approximately 30 minutes. (Set a timer)

3. While muffins are baking-make a batch of **yogurt**. Page 155.

4. Assemble **cookie dough** and start baking them (set a timer!) Page 154.

5. While cookies are baking. Make **chili relleno casserole**: Mix well 6 eggs, 1/4 cup yogurt, salt and pepper to taste; lay 1 can whole green chilies (seeded) and flattened out in bottom of buttered 9" by 9" pan, top with thin slices Monterey Jack cheese, add another can green chilies and a layer of cheddar cheese slices. Top with egg mixture and bake for 20-30 minutes at 350 degrees or until done. If you like salsa it's easy to find fresh types made without sugar or make your own using chopped tomato, onion, a little bit of jalapeno, cilantro, salt and a squeeze of fresh lemon or lime.

6. Make a simple **meatloaf** –we like 1 egg, finely chopped onion, garlic, tomatoes, grated zucchini, salt and pepper in ours. Place in bread pan and put in oven at 350 for 1 hour or until meat is fully cooked in the center.

7. Place **chicken** pieces (with skin on) in baking pan. Add salt, pepper and any other spices you'd like. Bake with the meatloaf approximately 1 hour.

8. Wash your hands well after handling raw chicken then assemble in a large bowl with a lid, a large **salad of greens** (we use at least a ½ head), celery, carrots, red cabbage, and radishes. This is your base salad you can pull from during the week. We usually make enough for 4 days worth of salads then make more. Garnish individual salads with additional vegetables before eating, as green peppers, tomatoes, cucumbers and avocado don't last very long once cut up.

9. Make a simple yet delicious **salad dressing**. Combine ½ cup olive oil, 6 Tablespoons white wine vinegar, 2 teaspoons stone-ground mustard, 1 clove garlic (pressed or minced), ½ t salt and ¼ t pepper.

10. Make a batch of **butternut squash fries**. See page 153.

11. Pour yourself another glass of wine, kick up your feet and eat a lovely dinner knowing you have prepared and tucked away many meals for the week ahead. You should have a lovely choice of chicken or meatloaf, a side salad with dressing, and winter squash fries. Top this off with a freshly baked muffin or cookie and a pat on the back!

For the week ahead your meal choices could include:

Breakfast:

-Yogurt with blueberries, honey, and walnuts

-Muffins

-Chili Rellenos

-Cheeseburger Omelet (using a slice of meatloaf crumbled in your eggs and some cheese)

-Chicken sausages

-Fresh fruit, fruit juice, yogurt and honey (blended into a smoothie)

Lunch:

-Green salad with chicken and avocado

-Chili rellenos and green salad

-Chicken soup and a muffin

-Yogurt, fruit, nuts and muffins

Dinners:

-Meat loaf with green beans and winter squash

-Baked chicken with broccoli and salad

-Chili Rellenos with salsa, steamed broccoli or

-Cauliflower, green salad

-Chicken soup, salad, muffins

-Chicken sausages baked in sauerkraut, green beans

Snacks:

-Fresh fruit

-Cookies and muffins

-Fruit and yogurt smoothies

-Mixed nuts and raisins

-Fried Cheese

-Fruit and cheese platter (assemble various cheeses, grapes, dried figs, apricots, sliced apples, and walnut halves on a plate)

-Steamed broccoli and cauliflower with grated cheese sprinkled on top

As you can see, you have created many choices for meals during the week by preparing and cooking ahead. Keep in mind this is just an example of how to manage your cooking chores especially if time is at a premium. As you become more comfortable with what foods are on the legal list, branch out and cook pizzas, breads, nachos, maybe more exotic fare you invent by substituting ingredients in your own family recipes.

Here's to your good health!

Reference Page

1. Warner Chilcott -2010 News-Medical.Net-
   http://www.news-medical.net/news/20100507/Warner-
   Chilcott-reports-209525-increase-in-first-quarter-2010-
   revenues.aspx
2. Salix Pharmaceuticals Reports 1Q2008 Results-
   http://www.salix.com
3. Crohn's Disease - Pipeline Assessment and Market Forecasts
   to 2017-www.marketresearch.com
4. http://www.ccfa.org/info/about/ucp
5. http://www.webmd.com
6. http://www.ccfa.org/about/news/scd
7. http://www.scdiet.org/6research/
8. Gottschall, E. (2004). *Breaking the vicious cycle: intestinal
   health through diet*. Baltimore, Ontario: Kirkton Pr Ltd.

Two Steps Forward, One Step Back

~A Journey Through Life~Ulcerative Colitis

And The Specific Carbohydrate Diet

By Tucker Sweeney & Carol Thompson (2011)

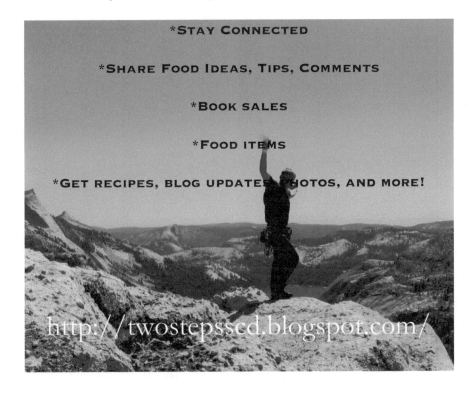

*STAY CONNECTED

*SHARE FOOD IDEAS, TIPS, COMMENTS

*BOOK SALES

*FOOD ITEMS

*GET RECIPES, BLOG UPDATES, PHOTOS, AND MORE!

http://twostepsscd.blogspot.com/